The Essential
DIABETIC
COOKBOOK
FOR BEGINNERS

TABLE OF CONTENT

INTRODUCTION FOR DIABETIC COOKBOOK FOR BEGINNERS 5

WHAT IS DIABETIC? 5

WHAT ARE THE ADVANTAGES OF A DIABETIC COOKBOOK? 6

DIETARY TIPS FOR DIABETICS? 7

GUIDELINE FOR DIABETICS? 8

BREAKFAST RECIPES 11

1. Pear spiced oatmeal 11
2. Peanut butter and crisp bread 11
3. Avocado egg toast 12
4. Cherry smoothie 13
5. shakshuka 14
6. Mago raspberry smoothie 14
7. Scrambled egg with sausage 15
8. Classic omelet and green 15
9. Tofu scrambled 15
10. Banana porridge 16
11. Vegan popcorn 16
12. Cottage cheese bowls 17
13. Quake and cucumber toast 17
14. Bean and bacon breakfast tacos 18
15. Pumpkin protein pancakes 19
16. Berry yoghurt bowl 19
17. Almond energy bowls 19
18. Trail mix hot cereal 20
19. Pineapple and grapefruit detox 20
20. Lance French toast 21

PORK BEEF AND LAMB RECIPE 22

1. Lamb mushroom cheeseburger 22
2. Pork loin, carrot and gold tomato roast 22
3. Autumn pork chops 23
4. Beef stroganoff 24
5. Ritzy beef stew 25
6. Pulled pork sandwich with Apricot jelly 26
7. Parmesan Golden pork chops 26
8. Beef picadillo 27
9. Pork souvlakia with tzatziki sauce 28
10. Roasted beef with shallot sauce 29
11. Pork Diane 29
12. Steak with brained mushroom 30

13. Sloppy Joes 31
14. Citrus pork tenderloin 31
15. Asian beef bowls 32
16. Bacon and cauliflower casserole 32
17. Cajun beef and rice skillet 33
18. Steak Sandwich 33
19. Easy lamb cutlets 34
20. Ham and brie turnovers 35

POULTRY RECIPES 35

1. Turkey cabbage soup 35
2. Speedy chicken cacciatore 36
3. Chicken Provencal 36
4. Wine-poached chicken with herbs and vegetables. 37
5. Turkey with almond duxelles 37
6. One pan chicken dinner 39
7. Spicy chicken drumsticks 39
8. Thanksgiving turkey breast 40
9. Chicken Caesar salad 41
10. Taco stuffed sweet potato. 43
11. Rosemary chicken with potatoes and beans ..43
12. Chicken with lemon caper pan sauces 44
13. Italian chicken thighs 44
14. Spicy cacciatore 45
15. Chicken wings with parmesan sauce 45
16. Chicken fajitas 46
17. Chicken shawarma 47
18. Turkey schnitzel 48
19. Chicken quesadillas 48
20. Chicken lettuce wraps 49

VEGETABLES AND SIDE DISHES RECIPE 50

1. Fresh dill dip 50
2. Instant popcorn 50
3. Radish chip 51
4. Quinoa and white bean loaf 51
5. Roasted veggies bowl 52
6. Veggies fajitas 53
7. Roasted asparagus 54
8. Butternut squash soup 54
9. Cauliflower tots 54
10. Garlic herb sweet potato fries 55
11. Zucchini fritter 56
12. Onion rings 56

13. STUFFED BELL PEPPERS 57

14. KALE CHIPS 58

15. COLD SESAME CUCUMBER NOODLE SALAD 58

16. CARROT STICKS WITH PESTO...................................59

17. CARRIED BROCCOLI WITH CHILI AND LEMON ZEST 60

18. GARLIC SAUTEED SPINACH WITH PINE NUTS.............60

19. PUMPKIN SEEDS CLUSTERS...................................60

20. JICAMA CARROT AND APPLE SALAD 61

DESSERT RECIPES 61

1. ORANGE SORBET 61

2. FRUIT MOUSSE 62

3. KETO ALMOND FLOUR CROISSANTS..........................62

4. PEACH SMOOTHIE 63

5. BANANA CHOCOLATE BITES...................................65

6. LEMON TART 65

7. BAKED APPLE WITH ORANGE 66

8. COCONUT FLOUR MUFFINS 67

9. FRUIT AND NUTS WITH SEEDS 67

10. NUT AND FRUIT ROLL...68

11. COTTAGE CHEESE BAKED RAISINS 68

12. ALMOND COOKIES 69

13. OAT BARS WITH NUTS AND DRIED FRUIT 69

14. TIRAMISU SHOTS 70

15. BRULE ORANGE 71

16. BROILED STONE FRUIT 72

17. KAMUT PORRIDGE 72

18. COCONUT PUDDING CLOUD 73

19. PINEAPPLE FROZEN YOGHURT...............................73

20. BLUEBERRY LEMON CUPCAKE 73

Title: "The Diabetic Cookbook for Beginners: Delicious Recipes for Managing Diabetes and Enjoying Flavorful Meals"

Introduction:

Welcome to "The Diabetic Cookbook for Beginners," your comprehensive guide to delicious, diabetes-friendly cooking. Whether newly diagnosed or seeking to better manage your condition, this cookbook is your roadmap to enjoying flavorful meals while supporting your health and well-being.

Living with diabetes presents unique challenges, but it doesn't mean you have to sacrifice taste or culinary enjoyment. With the right knowledge, ingredients, and recipes, you can create meals that are tasty, healthy, and supportive of your diabetes management goals.

In this cookbook, we've curated a collection of easy-to-follow recipes designed for beginners. Each recipe is crafted with care to ensure it meets the dietary guidelines for managing diabetes while delivering taste and satisfaction. Whether you're cooking for yourself, your family, or your friends, these recipes will inspire you to explore the world of diabetic-friendly cuisine with confidence and creativity.

We aim to empower you to take control of your health through the foods you eat. By making informed choices and embracing wholesome, nutrient-rich ingredients, you can support your body's needs and maintain stable blood sugar levels. With our cookbook as your guide, you'll discover that managing diabetes can be both delicious and rewarding.

In addition to mouthwatering recipes, "The Diabetic Cookbook for Beginners" provides essential information and practical tips to help you navigate your culinary journey. From understanding carbohydrates and portion control to mastering cooking techniques and ingredient substitutions, we're here to support you every step of the way.

Whether craving comforting classics, adventurous flavors, or satisfying sweets, you'll find something to delight your taste buds in this cookbook. From hearty breakfasts and satisfying lunches to flavorful dinners and indulgent desserts, we've got you covered with recipes that prioritize taste, health, and simplicity.

Starting a new dietary journey can feel overwhelming, but we're here to make it easy and enjoyable. With our beginner-friendly approach and expert guidance, you'll soon discover the joy of cooking and eating well with diabetes.

So, grab your apron, preheat your oven, and embark on a delicious adventure together. Welcome to "The Diabetic Cookbook for Beginners" – where every meal celebrates health, flavor, and possibility.

Here's to good food, good health, and good living!

What is Diabetic?

The term "diabetic" describes a person whose blood sugar levels are consistently high due to a chronic medical disease known as diabetes. When someone is said to be "diabetic," it implies they have the disease and are taking steps to control it, such as eating right, exercising, and keeping an eye on their blood sugar levels.

Insulin is a hormone that balance blood sugar levels; diabetes increase when the body does not make enough insulin or its cells resist its effects. The consequence is high blood sugar, which, if unchecked, can cause various health problems.

Diabetes comes in many forms, including:

Diabetic Fever: This kind develops when the pancreatic beta cells responsible for generating insulin are wrongly targeted and killed by the immune system. Insulin therapy is a lifetime need for people with type 1 diabetes to balance their blood sugar levels.

The most prevalent kind of diabetes, type 2, is linked to unhealthy lifestyle choices, including being overweight, not having enough exercise, and eating poorly. Cells develop insulin resistance, and the pancreas may fail to secrete enough insulin to counteract this in type 2 diabetes. Adjustments to one's way of life, together with medicine and, in rare instances, insulin treatment, can help keep type 2 diabetes under control.

When insulin production is inadequate to satisfy the body's increased needs during pregnancy, a form of diabetes known as gestational diabetes develops. Although most women feel better after giving birth, it might raise the chance of getting type 2 diabetes in the future.

Extra Formats: Additional types of diabetes can develop as a result of certain medical or genetic factors; these include secondary diabetes and monogenic diabetes.

Being "diabetic" entails dealing with the day-to-day difficulties of controlling one's blood sugar levels, leading a healthy lifestyle, and avoiding or dealing with diabetes-related problems. It calls for a preventative strategy for health and wellness, often including seeing a doctor, keeping tabs on blood sugar levels, eating right, exercising frequently, and taking medicine as directed.

What are the advantages of a Diabetic cookbook?

People with diabetes can benefit greatly from using a diabetic cookbook. The main advantages are as follows:

Diabetic cookbooks contain healthy recipes that are adapted to the unique dietary requirements of people with diabetes. These recipes aim to assist with glucose control, general health, and the prevention of diabetes-related problems.

Carbohydrate, protein, fat, and fiber levels are just some of the nutritional details provided by diabetic recipes. People may use this data to better control their diabetes by making educated decisions about what they eat.

Well-Balanced meals: Diabetic cookbooks are all about helping you make nutritious, nutrient-dense meals that include lean meats, whole grains, veggies, fruits, and healthy fats. Maintaining this equilibrium is beneficial to health since it stabilizes blood sugar levels.

Portion management: A key component of controlling blood sugar levels and keeping a healthy weight is focusing on portion management in many diabetic recipes. People with diabetes can benefit from these cookbooks since they provide recipes with reasonable serving sizes, which makes it easier to regulate food intake.

Delicious and Diverse Options: Despite common misconceptions, diabetic-friendly meals don't have to be bland. People with diabetes may eat a diverse and delicious diet thanks to the abundance of tasty recipes found in diabetic cookbooks, which include everything from comfort meals to sweets and other cuisines.

Cookbooks for people with diabetes typically include instructional material on managing the disease, proper nutrition, meal planning, cooking methods, and recipes. By following this advice, people with diabetes can better control their condition and eat healthily.

To make recipes lower in carbs, sugars, and fats, diabetic cookbooks may include ingredient replacements. People can still eat the meals they love even though they have to watch what they eat because of these alternatives.

Recipes that the Whole Family Can Enjoy: A large number of diabetic cookbooks provide dishes that are suitable for both the diabetic and their loved ones. This promotes a welcoming and inclusive dining atmosphere by ensuring everyone can share healthy and tasty meals.

Preparing Meals: Diabetic cookbooks typically provide grocery lists, suggestions for batch cooking, and recommendations for meal planning to assist people with diabetes save time and effort while making their meals. This facilitates the achievement of dietary objectives and the maintenance of consistent eating patterns in patients with diabetes.

At their core, diabetic cookbooks provide people with diabetes more agency over their dietary health. These cookbooks empower people with diabetes to take charge of their health and live the life they want by offering evidence-based information, tasty recipes, and practical tools.

Dietary tips for diabetics?

One of the most important aspects of successfully controlling diabetes is dietary management. People who suffer from diabetes should follow these dietary guidelines:

Prioritize Carbohydrates:

Carbohydrates are the mandatory food group that affects blood sugar levels, so watch what you eat. Eat more complex carbs like beans, fruits, vegetables, and whole grains; they take longer to digest and bring about a more gradual spike in blood sugar.

Keep an eye on serving sizes:

For better glycemic control and calorie management, watch portion sizes. Always use measuring cups, food scales, or eye-level indicators to be sure you're eating the right amount.

Option for Foods with a Low Glycemic Index:

For a less pronounced impact on blood sugar levels, go for low glycemic index (GI) meals. Produce that isn't starchy, beans, whole grains, and most fruits fall into this category.

To assist in regulating blood sugar levels and induce fullness, include lean protein sources in your meals. Cut off the fat and consume lean meats, skinless chicken, fish, tempeh, lentils, and low-fat dairy.

Healthy Fats: Incorporate moderate amounts of heart-healthy fats like avocados, nuts, seeds, olives, and olive oil into your diet. These lipids can aid both insulin sensitivity and cardiovascular health.

Fruits, vegetables, whole grains, beans, nuts, and seeds are all great sources of fiber, so make sure you eat lots of them. Digestive slowdown, blood sugar regulation, and satiety enhancement are all benefits of a high-fiber diet.

Keep Sugar and Sweets to a Minimum:

Reducing your intake of sugary drinks, desserts, sweets, and sweetened snacks is a good place to start. Choose sugar-free products or fruits that are naturally sweet.

Keep Yourself Hydrated: To keep yourself hydrated, drink lots of water throughout the day. Blood sugar levels might fluctuate, so it's best to cut out on sugary drinks and alcohol.

When and How Much to Eat:

Maintaining regular meal times and spacing might aid with glucose regulation. Try eating smaller, more frequent snacks to avoid dangerous swings in blood sugar levels.

Avoid Hypoglycemia (low blood sugar) by drinking alcohol moderately and with meals if you must partake. Keep in mind that alcohol can make it harder to maintain your blood sugar levels, which could mean that you need to make some changes to how you manage your diabetes.

Food Label Reading:

The carbohydrate amount, portion size, and total calories of food should be checked by reading the labels. Sugar and carbs may lurk in unexpected places in processed and packaged meals.

Consistent Exercise:

Make exercise a regular part of your regimen for better insulin sensitivity, lower blood sugar levels, and weight management. Try to work out both your aerobic and strength systems.

Think about Collaborating with an Accredited Dietician: Think about collaborating with an accredited dietician who focuses on diabetes care. You may get tailored nutritional guidance, assistance in developing a food plan, and encouragement to reach your health objectives from them.

Keep in mind that each person with diabetes is unique and that strategies that help some may have no effect on others at all. Control a close eye on your blood sugar levels, pay attention to your body, and communicate with your healthcare team to make any necessary modifications to your food and lifestyle.

Guideline for diabetics?

Diet, exercise, medication management, and monitoring are only a few lifestyle components covered in diabetes treatment guidelines. In general, people with diabetes should follow these guidelines:

Preventative Medical Exams: To monitor your blood sugar levels, evaluate your general health, and make any necessary adjustments to your treatment plan, schedule frequent check-ups with your healthcare practitioner.

Follow your healthcare provider's orders about monitoring your blood sugar levels. Regular monitoring allows you to learn your body's reactions to various meals, activities, and drugs.

Proper Dosage: If insulin or other prescription medicine is to be used, do it exactly as advice. Carefully adhere to all directions given by your healthcare provider. It is important to be mindful of the possibility of drug interactions and negative effects.

Have a vary diet rich in fruits, vegetables, whole grains, lean meats, and nutritionist fats to balance good health. Watch your carbohydrate consumption and portion sizes.

Managing weight, lowering the risk of cardiovascular problems, improving insulin sensitivity, and balancing blood sugar levels may all be achieved by regular physical activity. Two or more days a week should be devoted to muscle-strengthening exercises and 150 minutes of moderate-intensity aerobic activity.

Weight management entails keeping the weight down or becoming in the best shape of your life by prioritizing good food and regular exercise. A better ability to regulate blood sugar and a decreased risk of complications from diabetes can be achieved with even a modest weight loss.

Stress Management: To keep blood sugar levels under control, it is recommended to use stress-reduction strategies such as deep breathing, meditation, yoga, or mindfulness.

If you smoke, it's important to find help to stop. In addition to growing the risk of cardiovascular disease and diabetic complications, smoking makes both conditions worse.

Reducing Alcohol Use: Drink alcohol sparingly and with meals if you so choose. Alcohol can interfere with diabetic drugs and alter blood sugar levels.

Take good care of your feet by checking them daily for infections, blisters, and sores. Foot problems are more likely in people with diabetes since the disease can reduce blood flow and nerve sensitivity in the feet.

Scheduling frequent dental and vision exams: The best way to find and avoid diabetic eye issues is to check your eyes regularly. Gum disease is more common among diabetics; thus, it's important to get frequent dental checkups and cleanings.

Training and Assistance: Learn as much as possible about diabetes care through books, online forums, and in-person workshops. You can take charge of your health and make educated decisions when you have all the information regarding your situation.

Prepare for the Unexpected: Know how to handle situations with low or high blood sugar or Hypoglycemia if you have diabetes. Always have glucose pills or insulin, and know when to seek medical assistance.

Consistent Sleep: Make sure you receive adequate sleep every night. Not getting enough sleep can affect your health in general and your blood sugar levels in particular. Get between seven and nine hours of good sleep every night.

Recognizing Medical Alerts: Make sure others know you have diabetes by wearing a medical alert necklace or bracelet. In an emergency, this might be useful as you cannot express your medical status verbally.

These recommendations provide a framework for efficient diabetes management and complication risk reduction. But, to achieve your unique objectives while managing diabetes, it is critical to collaborate closely with your healthcare team. Successful diabetes control requires proactive self-care, regular contact

with healthcare providers, and adherence to
prescribed medicines.

1. Pear spiced oatmeal

Prep time: 10 min

Cook time: 20 min

Total time: 30 min

Serving: 2

INGREDIENTS

- 1/2 tbsp coconut oil
- 1 small pear, finely chopped
- 1/2 tsp cinnamon
- 1/4 tsp cardamom
- 1/4 tsp nutmeg
- pinch of salt
- 1 cup of unsweetened almond milk (or milk of choice
- 1 cup of water
- 3/4 cup of rolled oats
- 2 tbsp steel-cut oats, *see note
- 2 tbsp ground flax seeds
- 1 tbsp chia seeds
- 2 tbsp maple syrup
- 1 tsp vanilla extract
- Spiced Pear Topping
- 1 pear, chopped
- 1/2 tbsp coconut oil
- 1/2 tsp cinnamon
- 1/4 tsp cardamom
- 1/4 tsp nutmeg
- 1 tbsp maple syrup

INSTRUCTIONS

1. Heat an average saucepan over medium heat and add the coconut oil. Once heated, sauté the pear pieces in a mixture of salt, spices, and finely chopped pear for 5 minutes or until the pears have softened. Mix the milk and water in a saucepan. Next, add the oats, chia seeds, and flax seeds. Stir until well combined. Reduce heat to medium-low and simmer oats for 10 to 15 minutes or until they absorb most of the liquid and become thick.

2. Put the coconut oil in a small pan over medium heat to prepare the spicy pear topping. Toss in the pears and seasonings after they're heated.

3. Once the pears begin to soften, which should take around three to five minutes, reduce the heat to medium-low. Once the pears caramelize in the syrup, add the maple syrup and continue cooking until they soften even more. Take off the stove and place aside.

4. Put the maple syrup and vanilla extract into the saucepan after the oats have cooked for a few minutes. Arrange the spiced pears on top of the portions in the serving dishes.

2. Peanut butter and crisp bread

Prep time: 20 min

Cook time: 30 min

Total time: 40 min

Serving: 3

INGREDIENTS

- Crispbread with peanut butter & chia
- 1/2 cup of sunflower seeds
- 1/2 cup of hazelnuts
- 1/2 cup of sesame seeds

- 1/2 cup almond flour (buckwheat flour is also ok)
- 3 tbsp chia seeds
- 3/4 cup of water
- 2 tbsp peanut butter
- 0,75 tsp salt

INSTRUCTIONS

1. Prepare the oven for 175°C (350°F).
2. After adding the chia seeds to the water, let them sit for 20 minutes.
3. The hazelnuts should be finely chopped using a knife or food processor.
4. Gather all of the components in a big, roomy bowl. Mix thoroughly. Use your hands to squirm if necessary. A thick dough has been formed.
5. To line your baking pans, cut two pieces of parchment paper to size.
6. Grease or melt the butter and brush it onto the parchment papers.
7. Split the dough in half and divide it evenly among the two sheets of paper. Roll out each half of the dough as thin as you can using your hands, making sure to use your fingers to repair any tears that may occur. To get a flawless finish, you may also use a spatula.
8. Top with flaky sea salt.
9. Ten minutes in the oven should do the trick.
10. Take the crisp bread out of the oven and carefully turn it over.
11. After 15 minutes, take out the parchment paper and return the bread to the oven to toast until it becomes dry and crisp. Depending on the thickness of the dough, the cooking time will vary.
12. Keep the bread in the oven until it gets crisp and dry, even if it's a little mushy in the center.

3. Avocado egg toast

Prep time: 3 min

Cook time: 7 min

Total time: 10 min

Serving: 1

INGREDIENTS

- ¼ avocado seeded and peeled
- 1 slice whole grain bread or bread of choice
- Sea salt to taste
- Freshly cracked black pepper to taste
- Fried Eggs
- ½ tbsp butter
- 1 large egg
- Scrambled Eggs
- ½ tbsp butter
- 2 eggs
- Boiled Eggs
- 2 eggs
- Poached Eggs
- 2 tsp white vinegar
- 1 large egg

INSTRUCTIONS

1. After the bread is toasted in the toaster until golden and crisp, spread the quarter avocado on top of the toast and top it with slices of mashed avocado. Sprinkle with salt and pepper and top with eggs or anything you choose.
2. To cook the eggs in a frying pan, melt the butter in a skillet over

average-high heat. Quickly lower the heat to low after cracking the egg onto the skillet. After around 7 to 10 minutes of cooking without cover, the whites should be fully set, and the yolks should be thick enough to your taste.

3. Preheat the butter in a nonstick pan over average-high heat for the scrambled eggs. In a small dish, whisk the eggs. Carefully pour the mixture into the center of the pan. After the sides begin to set, carefully fold the eggs in half to cook them all the way through, which should take about two or three minutes.

4. Put the eggs in a pot and bring to a boil. Submerge the eggs completely in cold water by pouring it over them. Reduce the heat to low and boil the water for 4 minutes for soft, 6 minutes for medium, and 12 minutes for hard, or until done according to your preference. Get a basin of cold water ready. Once the eggs are fried, place them in the ice water bath to cool entirely before peeling.

5. A big saucepan of boiling water is all needed to poach eggs. Break one egg into a little dish. Combine the vinegar and water, then whip up a whirlpool with the hot water. Turn the heat down low enough so the water boils rapidly at the pot's base. After that, gently place the egg in the saucepan's center and cook for three to four minutes or until it reaches the doneness you choose. Use a spoon to remove the egg.

4. Cherry smoothie

Prep time: 5 min

Total time: 5 min

Serving: 2

INGREDIENTS

- 1 cup of unsweetened almond milk
- ¼ cup of Greek yogurt
- 1 ½ cups of cherries pitted and frozen (10 oz)
- 1 banana frozen
- ½ tsp pure vanilla extract
- 1 tbsp honey
- Optional add-ins
- 1 scoop protein powder (vanilla or chocolate)
- 1 cup of spinach
- 1 tbsp chia seeds
- ¼ tsp cinnamon

INSTRUCTIONS

1. Place items in the container in the sequence shown. Use a Vitamix or similar high-powered blender.
2. Put the cover on and blend for 50-60 seconds, starting at low speed and rising to high, or until the mixture is smooth.
3. Shake well and serve in four glasses.

5. shakshuka

Prep time: 5 min

Cook time: 20 min

Total time: 25 min

Serving: 4

INGREDIENTS

- 1 brown onion, thickly sliced
- 500g pkt Coles Australian Tri Color Capsicum, halved, seeded, thinly sliced
- 2 x 400g cans diced tomatoes
- 4 Coles Australian Free-Range Eggs
- 1/2 cup of flat-leaf parsley leaves

INSTRUCTIONS

Turn the heat up to medium-high in a big, nonstick skillet. Sauté the capsicum and onion for 5 minutes, stirring periodically, until the onion softens.

Stir in the tomato and continue cooking for another five minutes until the sauce boils and thickens slightly.

Indent the tomato mixture four times with the back of a spoon. Put one egg into each depression carefully. Turn the heat down to low. To achieve soft yolks or desired doneness, partially cover and cook for 10 minutes. Serve garnished with a sprig of parsley.

6. Mago raspberry smoothie

Prep time: 10 min

Total time: 10 min

Serving: 4

INGREDIENTS

- 12 oz mangoes (peeled, pit removed, cut into chunks)
- 8 oz raspberries (frozen)
- 3 tbsp honey
- 1 tsp lemon juice
- 1 tbsp chia seeds
- 1/2 cup whole milk
- 8 mint leaves (divided)
- 2 cups ice

INSTRUCTIONS

1. Stir together all of the components: Add 2 cups of ice, 12 ounces of mangoes, 8 ounces of frozen raspberries, 3 tablespoons of honey, 1 teaspoon of lemon juice, 1 tablespoon of chia seeds, 1/2 cup of whole milk, and 4 mint leaves to a blender. Blend until smooth.
2. Making a Mango Raspberry Smoothie, Step One
3. Until smooth, blend for 30 seconds.
4. smoothie made of pink fruit in a pitcher
5. Dispense into glasses for serving.
6. Part 2: A Mango Raspberry Smoothie Recipe
7. Present with a garnish: Separate the smoothie into four equal portions and serve. Before serving, top with the remaining four mint leaves.

7. Scrambled egg with sausage

Prep time: 5 min

Cook time: 10 min

Total time: 15 min

Serving; 4

INGREDIENTS

- 6 links of pork sausage
- 6 large eggs
- ¾ cup of milk
- ¾ cup of shredded sharp Cheddar cheese

INSTRUCTIONS

1. Sauté the sausage in a big, deep pan. Brown all sides while cooking over medium-high heat. After draining, cut into small pieces and lay aside.
2. Combine the milk and eggs and whip them while the sausage is cooking. Transfer eggs to a skillet. Before the eggs are set, stir in the cheese. Before serving, heat and combine with sausage.

8. Classic omelet and green

Prep time: 10 min

Cook time: 10 min

Total time: 20 min

Serving: 3

INGREDIENTS

- 3 Tbsp olive oil, divided
- 1 yellow onion, finely chopped
- 8 large eggs
- Kosher salt
- 2 Tbsp butter
- 1 oz Parmesan, finely grated
- 2 Tbsp fresh lemon juice
- 3 oz baby spinach

INSTRUCTIONS

1. Set a big nonstick pan over medium heat and add 1 tablespoon of oil. Sauté the onion for 6 minutes or until it becomes soft, stirring periodically. Move to a bowl.
2. In a big basin, mix the eggs with 1 tbsp of water and half a tsp of salt. Melt the butter by returning the skillet to the medium heat. While swirling continuously with a rubber spatula, fry the eggs until they are almost set. Reduce heat to low and cover pan firmly; stay cooking for another 4 to 5 minutes or until eggs are almost set.
3. Before folding in half, sprinkle sautéed onion and Parmesan on top.
4. Combine the leftover 2 tablespoons of olive oil and lemon juice in a middle bowl and whisk. Arrange the omelet on a bed of spinach and drizzle with vinaigrette.

9. Tofu scrambled

Prep time: 5 min

Cook time: 10 min

Total time: 15 min

Serving: 3

INGREDIENTS

- 1 tbsp olive oil
- (1) 16-ounce block firm tofu
- 2 tbsp nutritional yeast
- 1/2 tsp salt, or more to taste
- 1/4 tsp turmeric
- 1/4 tsp garlic powder

- 2 tbsp non-dairy milk, unsweetened and unflavored

INSTRUCTIONS

1. Put the olive oil in a skillet and set it over medium heat. Mash the tofu block in the same pan using a potato masher or a fork. Add it to the pan by crumbling it with your hands. Tofu will release most of its water when cooked for 3–4 minutes with frequent stirring.
2. Season with salt, turmeric, and garlic powder, and then stir in the nutritional yeast. Stir occasionally while cooking for approximately 5 minutes.
3. Place in the soy milk and whisk to combine. Toast, steamed greens, avocado slices, spicy sauce, parsley, and other breakfast items can be served immediately.

10. Banana porridge

Prep time: 5 min

Cook time: 10 min

Total time: 15 min

Serving: 2

INGREDIENTS

- 150 g oats
- 1 banana
- 1 handful raisins
- 250 ml water
- 20 g walnuts
- 2 tsp. cinnamon

INSTRUCTIONS

1. After halving it lengthwise, chop the banana into slices that are approximately 1 cm thick.
2. Toss the oats with the banana and raisins in a saucepan.
3. Bring the water to a boil in a saucepan over medium heat. To avoid the mixture from sticking, stir it occasionally.
4. Reduce the heat to low after it begins to simmer. Simmer for approximately 10 minutes or until the banana is tender. Add a little water (or a milk substitute) if it becomes too dry. Cut the walnuts into little pieces while you wait.
5. Toss in the nuts and cinnamon after the porridge has been cooked.

11. Vegan popcorn

Prep time: 4 min

Cook time: 6 min

Total time: 10 min

Serving: 5

INGREDIENTS

- 2 tbsp nutritional yeast
- ¼ tsp smoked paprika
- ¼ tsp turmeric (optional)
- ½ tsp garlic powder or onion powder (optional)
- ½-1 tsp fine sea salt
- 2-3 tbsp coconut oil or vegan butter
- ⅓ cup of popping corn kernels

INSTRUCTIONS

1. Prepare a small bowl and combine nutritional yeast, smoked paprika, turmeric, garlic powder (if using), and salt. Remove from the heat.
2. The oil has to be heated for one minute over medium heat in a big saucepan until it melts.
3. Toss in three kernels of corn, cover with the lid, and shake the pot every

so often to disperse the kernels. The oil is ready when kernels pop. Take the corn out of the pot.

4. Put the cover back on the saucepan and add the remaining kernels. Ensure the popcorn doesn't burn by shaking it every 8 to 10 seconds while it pops. The corn should be (nearly!) fully popped after a 6-second interval between pops, at which point you may remove it from the fire.

5. Toss the popcorn with the seasonings while it's still in the saucepan, cover it, and shake it to combine. Clear a big dish and serve.

12. Cottage cheese bowls

Prep time: 5 min

Total time: 5 min

Serving: 1

INGREDIENTS

- ¾ cup of low-fat cottage cheese, I like Good Culture
- 2 tbsp minced chives or finely minced scallion greens divided
- Freshly ground black pepper
- ½ cup of sliced Persian cucumbers
- ½ medium bell pepper, seeded and chopped
- 10 halved grape tomatoes
- 1 tbsp chopped, roasted shelled pistachios
- Kosher salt

INSTRUCTIONS

1. Mix the cottage cheese, 1 tablespoon of chives, and pepper in a small dish. Season with pepper to taste.

2. Toss in the peppers, tomatoes, cucumbers, and 1 tablespoon of chives. Top with a sprinkle of pistachios and garnish with the remaining chives.

3. Season with pepper and salt to taste.

13. Quake and cucumber toast

Prep time: 10 min

Total time: 10 min

Serving: 4

INGREDIENTS

- 4 oz. (125g) cream cheese, room temperature
- 2 oz. (60g) feta cheese, room temperature
- 2 tbsp. green onion sliced
- ½ tsp. garlic minced
- 4 slices whole-grain bread toasted
- ½ cucumber sliced
- 2 radishes sliced
- ¼ cup of 10g alfalfa sprouts or other
- salt & black pepper

INSTRUCTIONS

1. Gather the cream cheese, feta, green onion, and garlic in a small bowl. Add salt and pepper as to your taste, then blend well.

2. Before you toast the bread, ensure each piece is uniformly coated with the cream cheese.

3. On top, arrange the sprouts, cucumber, and radishes. Add a little more pepper and salt and pepper to taste.

14. Bean and bacon breakfast tacos

Prep time: 10 min

Cook time: 15 min

Total time; 25 min

Serving: 4

INGREDIENTS

- 4 slices of thick-cut bacon, sliced (about 113g or 4oz total)
- Canned refried beans (1 15oz/425g can)
- Fresh lime juice (from 1 lime)
- Ground cumin
- Garlic powder
- Onion Powder
- Chili flakes
- Salt
- Cracked black pepper (to taste)
- Water
- White corn tortillas (4)
- Eggs (4)
- Chile crisp or sriracha
- Queso fresco crumbled
- Pickled red onions or jalapenos
- Fresh cilantro, chopped

INSTRUCTIONS

1. Cut the bacon into large, chunky pieces.
2. Sauté the bacon, covered, in a nonstick pan over medium-high heat. After the bacon has browned somewhat and released most of its fat, toss it about and let it crisp for another two or three minutes. It's done when it becomes crisp and a deep reddish brown color. Put on a platter lined with paper towels and set aside to drain.
3. While that's happening, bring the bacon pan back up to medium heat and heat a small nonstick sauté pan on low.
4. Put the refried beans in a dish that can be microwaved, cover with a moist paper towel, and cook for 2 minutes while the pan is heating.
5. Season the heated beans with ½ lime juice, ground cumin, garlic powder, onion powder, red chili flakes, salt, and cracked black pepper. Sprinkle with a teaspoon of powdered cumin. Add a little water if necessary and stir until the beans are combined into a creamy consistency. Before serving, check the seasoning with a taste.
6. To save some of the rendered bacon grease, fry the eggs in the same pan. The eggs will get a little more colorful and crispier on the bottom since you're cooking them rapidly.
7. Toss the eggs once the bottom becomes crispy and firm. On side 2, let the egg whites set just a bit. On the inside, the yolk should be somewhat runny and just beginning to set.
8. In the second pan, heat the tortillas over low heat.
9. Spread the refried beans over a tortilla that has been cooked. Top with ½ of the rendered crispy bacon, a fried egg, chili crisp, crumbled queso fresco, chopped fresh cilantro, and a few pickled red onions. Put the taco together.

15. Pumpkin protein pancakes

Prep time: 10 min

Cook time: 15 min

Total time: 25 min

Serving: 4

INGREDIENTS

- ½ cup of oatmeal
- ½ cup of plain, nonfat Greek yoghurt
- ½ cup of canned pumpkin
- 1 ½ tbsp zero-calorie brown sugar sweetener (Swerve brand)
- ½ cup of egg or liquid egg whites
- 1 tbsp flaxseed meal
- ¼ tsp cinnamon

INSTRUCTIONS

1. Put everything in a food processor or blender. The blender is the most effective tool for our task.
2. Process a smooth batter at high speed, stopping to scrape down sides and pulse as required.
3. Pound or heat a pan or skillet to 330–340°F. Alternatively, cook over medium-low heat in a skillet. Dip a little brush into the oil.
4. Before the edges dry, pour the batter into the pan and heat until little bubbles appear.
5. Cook until done, then turn over. Because the yoghurt gives these pancakes a particularly smooth and creamy texture, they might need a little more cooking time than regular pancakes.
6. With maple syrup and butter, or apple butter, it is served.

16. Berry yoghurt bowl

Prep time: 5 min

Total time: 5 min

Serving: 1

INGREDIENTS

2 cups of FAGE Total 0%, 2%, 5%

½ cup of strawberries, hulled and sliced

½ cup of raspberries

½ cup of blueberries

2 heaping tablespoons granola

Honey, maple syrup or agave

INSTRUCTIONS

1. Spoon one cup of yoghurt into every dish. Split the granola, raspberries, blueberries, and strawberries in half and put half into each bowl. Drizzle honey over the dishes.

17. Almond energy bowls

Prep time: 10 min

Total time: 10 min

Serving: 1

INGREDIENTS

- 1 cup of raw almonds
- ½ cup of almond butter
- ¼ cup of rice syrup (or maple syrup)

INSTRUCTIONS

2. Blend all of the elements in a food processor.
3. Form little balls out of the dough using a spoon.
4. To make the balls last all week, put them in an airtight container and keep them in the fridge or freezer.

18. Trail mix hot cereal

Prep time: 3 min

Cook time: 18 min

Total time: 21 min

Serving: 6

INGREDIENTS

- ½ cup of cashews
- ½ cup of peanuts
- 1 cup of corn Chex cereal
- 1 cup of pretzels
- 2 tbsp honey
- 2 tbsp Sriracha
- 1 tbsp neutral oil
- 1 tsp liquid aminos, or soy sauce
- Pinch of salt

INSTRUCTIONS

1. Heat the oven to 300 degrees.
2. A medium bowl should contain the Sriracha, honey, oil, and liquid aminos/soy sauce. Combine by whisking. Toss in the peanuts, cashews, pretzels, and Chex with the Sriracha-honey sauce, then stir to combine.
3. After lining a cooking sheet with parchment paper, spread the mixture evenly and season with salt.
4. Take out from the oven and let cool for approx. 18 minutes (check after 15 to ensure the mixture isn't burning; ovens differ).
5. Put the cooled mixture into bags with zip tops.

19.Pineapple and grapefruit detox

Prep time: 10 min

Total time: 10 min

Serving: 2

INGREDIENTS

- 1 cup of pineapple fresh or frozen
- 2 cups of kale or spinach leaves
- 1.5 inches ginger peeled
- 1 small lemon peeled
- 1/2 green apple
- 1 handful wheatgrass
- 1/2 cup of water or coconut water
- ice cubes

INSTRUCTIONS

1. Smoothly combine the following ingredients: spinach, ginger, apple, lemon, pineapple, and wheatgrass (if used). Half a cup of water or coconut water can be added if more liquid is required, which is common when using frozen pineapple instead of fresh.
2. You may adjust the smoothness by adding up to a cup of ice cubes and blending until smooth.
3. Graze on that detox smoothie!

20. Lance French toast

Prep time: 10 min

Cook time: 20 min

Total time: 30 min

Serving: 4

INGREDIENTS

- 4 large eggs
- 1 cup of 2% milk
- 2 tbsp sugar
- 1 tsp vanilla extract
- 1/4 tsp ground nutmeg
- 10 slices day-old French bread (3/4 inch thick)
- 1 to 2 tbsp butter
- Optional: Fresh berries and confectioners' sugar

INSTRUCTIONS

1. Whisk together the milk, eggs, sugar, vanilla, and nutmeg in a big basin. After greasing a 13x9-inch baking dish, set the bread inside. Add the egg mixture to the bread. Turn once to coat, then let soak for a few minutes. Thaw in the freezer. Before putting the slices back in the freezer, make sure they are airtight.

2. Warm up the oven to 450 degrees before baking. Scatter the frozen French toast pieces evenly over a cooking paper sheet that has been lightly oiled. Top with a few butter specks. Turn after 7 minutes and continue baking for another 10 to 12 minutes or until golden brown. Top with berries and garnish with confectioners' sugar if you want.

1. Lamb mushroom cheeseburger

Prep time: 20 min

Cook time: 20 min

Total time: 40 min

Serving: 1

INGREDIENTS

- 500g lamb mince
- 1 brown onion, grated
- 2 garlic cloves, crushed
- 3 tsp ground cumin
- 1 cup of stale breadcrumbs
- 1/4 cup of parsley leaves
- 3/4 cup of mint leaves, chopped
- 4 flat mushrooms, trimmed
- 3/4 cup Greek-style yoghurt
- 2 tbsp olive oil
- 4 hamburger buns, split
- Mixed salad leaves to serve
- 400g can beetroot slices, drained
- Vegetable crisps to serve

INSTRUCTIONS

1. Toss the lamb, garlic, onion, cumin, breadcrumbs, parsley, and half of the mint in a bowl. Toss with salt and pepper, then mix thoroughly. Cut into four equal patties. Reshape after pressing one mushroom into the center of each patty, stem side up. After transferring to a baking sheet, cover and chill for at least 30 minutes.
2. Mix the remaining mint with the yoghurt, add seasoning, and set aside until serving.
3. Heat a grill pan over medium heat. Drizzle oil over the patties on both sides. Grill the patties, mushroom side up, for 10 to 12 minutes, flip them over gently and grill for another 8 minutes or until done.
4. Warm up the rolls. Spread mint yoghurt on the bottom of the buns, then pile on the lamb patties, beets, salad greens, and salad toppings. Put the bread top on top of the sandwich with more yoghurt and veggie chips.

2. Pork loin, carrot and gold tomato roast

Prep time: 10 min

Cook time: 1hr

Total time: 1hr 10 min

Serving: 4

INGREDIENTS

- 3 pounds boneless pork loin roast
- 3 tbsp olive oil
- 4 cloves garlic, minced
- ½ tbsp dried crushed rosemary
- 1 tsp dried thyme
- 1 tsp dried oregano
- ½ tsp paprika
- 4 to 5 large carrots, peeled and cut into 1-inch pieces
- 4 stalks celery, cut into 1-inch pieces
- 1 pound baby Yukon gold potatoes, quartered
- sea salt, to taste
- freshly ground black pepper, to taste

INSTRUCTIONS

1. After removing the roast from the refrigerator, set it on a dish or work surface lined with parchment to

allow it to come to room temperature, fat side up.

2. Get the oven ready to bake at 450 degrees Fahrenheit while the roast is warming up.

3. Prepare a small bowl and combine the following ingredients: 1 tablespoon of olive oil, minced garlic, rosemary, thyme, oregano, and paprika. Stir to blend.

4. After the roast is at room temperature, make cross-hatch marks ¼ inch deep on the skin and fat, spaced 1 inch apart. While roasting, this will let the spice taste seep in.

5. Add a small amount of salt and pepper to the meat.

6. Put the beef in a baking dish with five quarts or more. Spread the herb mixture evenly over the pork loin and massage it in gently.

7. Place a piece of aluminum foil over the roast. Cook for the first twenty minutes.

8. Have the potatoes, celery, and carrots peeled and sliced. In a bowl, combine the vegetables with 1 tablespoon of olive oil, salt, and pepper. Set aside for now.

9. When the first 20 minutes of roasting are over, reduce the oven heat to 350°F and take the pork out.

10. Remove the foil and place the veggies on the pork roast in the dish. Season the pork and veggies with 1 more tablespoon of olive oil and scatter them on top.

11. After the pork roast reaches an internal temperature of 145°F and the veggies are soft, continue roasting uncovered at 350°F for another 35 to 45 minutes. Use a meat thermometer with an immediate read to find out when meat is done.

12. Take it out of the oven and put the foil back on again. Give it a 10-minute break.

13. Before slicing and serving the pork roast with the veggies, take it out of the oven and place it on a cutting board.

3. Autumn pork chops

Prep time: 20 min

Cook time: 25 min

Total time: 45 min

Serving: 3

INGREDIENTS

Topping:

- 1 small yellow onion, thinly sliced
- 1 cup of peeled and thinly sliced baking apples (preferably Cortland)
- 2 tbsp olive oil, or as needed
- 1 tbsp apple cider vinegar
- 2 tsp dried thyme
- 2 tsp dried rosemary
- 1 pinch brown sugar, or to taste

Pork Chops:

- 3 pork chops
- salt and ground black pepper to taste
- 1 pinch paprika, or more to taste
- 1 tbsp apple cider vinegar
- 1 tbsp olive oil

INSTRUCTIONS

1. Gently brown the onion and soften the apples, about 15 minutes, in a pan with 2 tbsp of olive oil, 1 tbsp of vinegar, thyme, and rosemary. To

taste, add brown sugar for sweetness. Remove from heat and set aside.

2. Salt, pepper, and paprika the pork chops and place them in a different skillet. Before you add the pork chops to the marinade, whisk together the vinegar and olive oil. The pork chops should be cooked for approximately 5 minutes on each side over medium heat or until the middle is no longer pink. When placed in the middle, an instant-read thermometer should register a temperature of at least 145 degrees Fahrenheit (63 degrees Celsius).

3. Place pork chops on a platter and garnish with the apple-onion mixture. Serve right away.

4. Beef stroganoff

Prep time: 10 min

Cook time: 35 min

Total time: 45 min

Serving: 4

INGREDIENTS

- 1 tbsp olive oil
- 1 onion, sliced
- 1 clove of garlic
- 1 tbsp butter
- 250g mushrooms, sliced
- 1 tbsp plain flour
- 500g fillet steak, sliced
- 150g crème fraiche
- 1 tsp English mustard
- 100ml beef stock
- ½ small pack of parsley, chopped

INSTRUCTIONS

1. Add 1 sliced onion to 1 tablespoon of olive oil in a nonstick skillet and sauté, stirring occasionally, over average heat until softened, about 15 minutes. If the onion sticks, add a splash of water.

2. Add 1 tablespoon of butter after crushing 1 garlic clove and cooking for another 2 to 3 minutes.

3. Add 250g of sliced mushrooms and simmer for about 5 minutes, or until softened, until the butter begins to froth.

4. After you've seasoned everything, transfer it to a dish.

5. Mix 1 tablespoon of ordinary flour with a little salt and pepper in a bowl. Coat 500 grams of sliced fillet steak with the flour mixture.

6. Fry the steak pieces for three to four minutes or until they are well browned, adding a splash of oil if the pan appears dry.

7. Toss the mushrooms and onions back into the skillet. Before adding to the pan, whisk together 150g crème fraiche, 1 teaspoon of English mustard, and 100ml of beef stock.

8. Cook over average heat for around 5 minutes.

9. Garnish with chopped parsley and eat with rice or pappardelle.

5. Ritzy beef stew

Prep time: 15 min

Cook time: 2hr 45 min

Total time: 3hr

Serving: 4

INGREDIENTS

- 1.2 kg / 2.4lb chuck beef, cut into 3.5 cm / 1.5" cubes
- 1 tsp each salt and pepper
- 3 tbsp olive oil, divided
- 1 large onion, halved, then cut into 1 cm / 2/5" slices
- 4 garlic cloves, minced
- 3 carrots, cut into 2.5cm / 1" pieces on the diagonal
- 2 celery stalks, cut into 2.5 cm / 1" pieces
- 1/3 cup / 50g flour
- 3 cups / 750ml beef broth/stock, salt reduced
- 2 cups / 500 ml red wine, bold and dry (Cab Sau, Burgundy, Merlot)
- 2 tsp Worcestershire Sauce
- 2 tbsp tomato paste
- 2 bay leaves, fresh or dried
- 4 sprigs thyme
- 400 g / 14 oz baby potatoes, halved
- More salt and pepper, to taste.

INSTRUCTIONS

1. Add salt and pepper to the meat.
2. Bring 1 1/2 tablespoons of oil to a smoking point in a big, heavy-bottomed casserole pot by heating it over high heat.
3. Toss a third of the steak and sear it well, approximately 4 minutes total. Put the meat in a basin and sear it again, adding additional oil if needed.
4. Lower the heat to a medium-high setting. Add 1 tablespoon of oil if needed. After 2 mins of cooking, add the garlic and onion and continue cooking till the onion softens and turns a little golden.
5. For a minute, toss the carrots and celery to coat them in the flavors.
6. Evenly distribute the flour over the surface, and then mix to coat.
7. Toss in the Worcestershire sauce, tomato paste, red wine, broth, and pasta. The tomato paste and flour should dissolve in the liquid when stirred.
8. Toss in the potato, bay leaf, thyme, cooked meat, and any juices. Stir. Make sure the water level covers everything, as seen in the video. If it doesn't, add a little more water.
9. Once it comes to a simmer, deduct the heat to low or medium-low and let it simmer softly.
10. Cook, covered, for 1 hour and 45 minutes, or until meat is almost tender; test at 1.5 hours with two forks.
11. After 30 minutes of simmering without the lid, the sauce should have reduced slightly. Watch the video to watch how the sauce should thicken into a thin gravy; at this point, the meat should be extremely soft.
12. Add salt and pepper as per your taste.
13. Top with mashed potatoes and garnish with parsley or a sprig of fresh thyme.

6. Pulled pork sandwich with Apricot jelly

Prep time: 10 min

Cook time: 10hr

Total time: 10hr 10 min

Serving: 8

INGREDIENTS

- 1 cup of barbecue sauce
- 1½ cups of apricot preserves
- 1-ounce dry onion soup mix 1 packet
- 2 tbsp Dijon Mustard
- 2 tbsp soy sauce
- 3-pound boneless pork shoulder roast
- 8 hamburger buns

INSTRUCTIONS

1. Gather all the ingredients in a medium bowl: barbecue sauce, apricot preserves, dry onion soup mix, Dijon mustard, and soy sauce.
2. Add the pork roast after spraying a slow cooker with nonstick cooking spray. Top the meat with the sauce.
3. Turn the heat down to low and simmer for 8 to 10 hours or up to 4 hours on high.
4. Use a slotted spoon to shred the meat, then top with buns or rolls.

7. Parmesan Golden pork chops

Prep time: 30 min

Cook time: 1hr 30 min

Total time: 2hr

Serving: 4

INGREDIENTS

FOR THE PORK CHOP

- 4 boneless pork chops, pounded thin (about 5 oz each)
- 3 eggs, beaten
- 2 cups flour
- 2 cups of panko bread crumbs
- 3 tbsp grated Parmesan cheese
- 3 tbsp clarified butter
- 8 slices provolone cheese

FOR THE TOMATO SAUCE

- 2 tbsp grapeseed oil
- 16 oz canned tomatoes
- 1 white onion, diced
- 8 cloves garlic minced
- 1 bunch basil; reserve ½ the bunch for garnish

FOR THE ORZO & SAUSAGE RAGOUT

- 2 lbs. ground spicy sausage
- 1 pt. orzo, cooked according to the package
- 4 cherry tomatoes, quartered
- 4 oz tomato sauce

INSTRUCTIONS

- Arrange three bowls. In the first, mix the all-purpose flour, pepper, and salt. Place the beaten eggs into the second bowl. Mixture the panko breadcrumbs and the Parmesan cheese in the third bowl.

- Sift flour over the cutlet on both sides. Egg wash is the next step. Finished last in the Parmesan and panko category. Remove from the heat.

CARROT SAUCE

- Sauté the garlic, onions, and grapeseed oil over medium heat.
- After 3 minutes of boiling, add the tomatoes. Bring to a low simmer.
- Third, while stirring occasionally, let the sauce boil for around half an hour.
- Place the sausage in a sauté pan and place it over medium-high heat. The sausage should be broken up using a spoon.
- Second, throw in the tomatoes. Just three more minutes of cooking time is required.
- Before setting away, stir in the tomato sauce.
- Get the oven preheated to 350 degrees.
- Place the breaded pork chop and clarified butter in a big pan and place it over medium heat.
- Cook the pork chop for approximately four minutes per side. You want your pork chops to be cooked thoroughly and golden brown.
- After that, set a baking sheet with the pork chops on it.
- Top each pork chop with a dollop of tomato sauce and two slices of provolone cheese.
- Melt the cheese by placing the pork chops in the oven for approximately three minutes.

- Spoon some tomato sauce into the middle of the platter and then add some orzo ragout on top.
- Top the ragout with the pork Parmesan. Sprinkle basil on top.

8. Beef picadillo

Prep time: 15 min

Cook time: 45 min

Total time: 1hr

Serving; 4

INGREDIENTS:

- 1 pound beef Top Sirloin Steak Boneless, cut 1 inch thick
- 1-1/2 teaspoons ground cumin
- 1 teaspoon dried oregano
- 1 tablespoon olive oil, divided
- 1 large all-purpose potato, peeled, cut into 1/2-inch chunks
- 1 medium onion, thinly sliced
- 1 medium green bell pepper, thinly sliced
- 1 can (15 ounces) tomato sauce
- 1/2 cup of raisins
- Serving Suggestions:
- Warmed flour tortillas or hot cooked rice, toasted sliced almonds, chopped fresh cilantro, sour cream (optional)

INSTRUCTIONS

- After halving the beef Top Sirloin Steak Boneless lengthwise, cut it crosswise into strips that are 1/8 to 1/4 inch thick. Combine the beef strips with the cumin and oregano in a medium bowl. Toss to coat.
- As an alternative to top sirloin steak, you can use one pound of beef flank steak or top round steak, both

of which should be sliced an inch thick.

- Get a big nonstick skillet heated over medium-high heat with 1 teaspoon of oil. After adding half of the beef, fry for 1–3 minutes, or until the meat's exterior is no longer pink. Take it out of the pan. Incorporate the leftover steak and an extra teaspoon of oil into the process. To taste, add salt; keep heated.

- Heat the leftover 1 teaspoon of oil in the same skillet over medium heat until it's hot. Sauté the onion, potato, and pepper. While stirring occasionally, cook for 5 minutes. Before boiling, stir in the raisins and tomato sauce. To soften the potato, reduce heat to low, cover, and boil gently for 15 to 18 minutes, stirring regularly. Before the steak is cooked completely, add it and simmer for another minute or two. Add more salt if needed.

- Toppings such as almonds, cilantro, and sour cream can be added to the beef mixture before serving it in tortillas or over hot cooked rice.

9. Pork souvlakia with tzatziki sauce

Prep time: 2hr

Cook time: 15 min

Total time: 2hr 15 min

Serving: 4

INGREDIENTS

- 4 bamboo skewers soaked in water for 30 mins.
- 1 lb. pork loin 1-inch cubed
- 1/2 cup extra virgin olive oil
- 4 tbsp. fresh lemon juice
- 2 tbsp. red wine vinegar
- 2 tbsp. chopped fresh oregano
- 2-3 garlic cloves grated
- 1/4 tsp. black pepper
- 1/4 tsp. salt

To serve…

- 2 pita flatbreads
- thinly sliced red onion
- diced fresh tomato
- fresh oregano sprigs

INSTRUCTIONS

1. In a zip-top bag, combine the pork cubes with the marinade ingredients. Submerge in the marinade for at least two hours, preferably all night.
2. Get the grill or pan hot over medium heat.
3. Skewer marinated pork cubes onto bamboo skewers that have been soaked. Reduce the marinade by boiling it in a small pot for two or three minutes.
4. To achieve a temperature of 160 degrees, use an instant-read thermometer and grill the skewers on each side for 2 minutes. After 5 minutes, set aside to cool.
5. "To serve..."
6. Arrange the skewers of pork souvlaki on top of the pita bread. Reduce the marinade and drizzle it over. Finish with a sprinkle of fresh oregano, chopped tomato, and thinly sliced red onion. On the side, a nutritious tzatziki sauce.

10. Roasted beef with shallot sauce

Prep time: 1 hr.

Cook time: 15 min

Total time: 1hr 15 min

Serving: 4

INGREDIENTS

- 3 lbs. Rocklands beef tri-tip, or any other roast, trimmed of some fat
- 1/4 lb. lean meat scraps or beef cubes
- 3 shallots, sliced
- Salt & pepper
- 1/2 bottle red wine (preferably an already opened bottle)
- 2 cups all-natural beef stock
- 2 cloves garlic, thinly sliced
- 3 sprigs rosemary

INSTRUCTIONS

1. Insert the rosemary and garlic into small cuts made in the meat. Make sure the meat is uniform in size throughout by tying it with twine.

2. Add salt and pepper to taste.

Third, heat the oil in a heavy Dutch oven and brown the meat on both sides. Bake at 325 to 350 degrees Fahrenheit, basting once every ten minutes with pan juices.

Cook until the internal temperature reaches 105-110 degrees Fahrenheit.

Set meat aside to rest for a third of the cooking time after removing heat.

As for the Slaw:

In a saucepan, bring the water to a boil. 1.

2. Add salt and pepper to the lean beef trimmings and brown them in heated fat. Take out the leftover meat and put it aside. Remove the pan from the heat, but be careful not to disturb the glaze that has formed at the bottom.

Add the red wine and sliced shallots to the pan, then scrape the top of the pan to deglaze it.

5. Add the reduced beef stock after the shallots and wine have been reduced nearly to dryness.

11. Pork Diane

Prep time: 10 min

Cook time; 35 mins

Total time: 45 min

Serving: 4

INGREDIENTS

- 1 tbsp water
- 1 tbsp white wine Worcestershire sauce
- 1 tsp lemon juice
- 1 tsp Dijon mustard
- 1 lb. boneless pork loin roast (cut into four 3/4- to 1-inch-thick slices)
- 1 tsp lemon-pepper seasoning
- 2 tbsp butter or 2 tablespoons margarine
- 1 tbsp snipped fresh chives or 1 tablespoon fresh parsley

INSTRUCTIONS

6. Mix the water, wine, Worcestershire sauce, lemon juice, and mustard in a small bowl. Set away.

7. Eliminate any fat that can be separated from the pork pieces.

8. Add a little lemon pepper on both sides of every slice.

9. While the pan is on medium heat, melt the butter.

10. Turn pork once throughout frying time and cook in hot butter for 6-10 minutes, or until the center is slightly pink and juices flow clear.

11. Take the meat out of the pan and set aside to reheat.

12. Take the pan off the heat and pour in the sauce. Stir until combined, making sure to scrape out any brown parts.

13. Spoon the sauce over the pork pieces and garnish with parsley or chives before serving.

12. Steak with brained mushroom

Prep time: 1hr 15 min

Cook time: 1hr

Total time: 2hr 15 min

Serving: 10

INGREDIENTS

- 2 tbsp canola oil
- 1 tbsp butter
- 4 cups of finely diced onions
- 2 large cloves garlic, crushed and peeled
- 2 tbsp tomato paste
- 2 tbsp sweet paprika
- 2 tsp chopped fresh marjoram, or 1 teaspoon dried
- 4 pounds beef chuck, trimmed and cut into 1 1/2-inch pieces
- 1 tsp salt, divided
- Freshly ground pepper, to taste
- 2 pounds cremini mushrooms, cut into 1/2-inch pieces
- 1 cup of reduced-sodium beef broth
- 8 large shiitake mushroom caps, cut into 1/2-inch pieces
- 2-3 tsp finely minced fresh tarragon, or dill for garnish

INSTRUCTIONS

1. Preheat the oven temperature to 350 grades Fahrenheit.

2. Smoothen the butter and oil in a heavy Dutch oven or large casserole pan over medium heat. Toss in the garlic and onions and sauté, turning occasionally, for 8 to 10 minutes, or until the onions are tender and starting to brown. Add the tomato paste, paprika, and marjoram and mix well.

3. Pepper the steak well and season it with half a teaspoon of salt. Carefully mix the cremini mushrooms with the meat in the saucepan. Toss in the broth and place a lid on top that fits snugly.

4. The meat should be extremely soft after 1 3/4 to 2 1/2 hours of baking. Remove the saucepan from the oven. After 15 minutes of covered baking, stir in the shiitake mushrooms. After removing it from the oven, cover it and allow it to rest untouched for around fifteen minutes.

5. Get rid of the fat in the stew by skimming or blotting it. Pour the mushrooms and meat into a bowl using a slotted spoon. Bring the saucepan back to a low simmer after removing it from the heat. Bring to a simmer until the sauce reaches a spoon-coating consistency. After approximately a minute of heating,

stir in the mushrooms, meat, and the remaining 1/2 teaspoon of salt to the sauce. If preferred, serve with a garnish of tarragon or dill.

13. Sloppy Joes

Prep time: 5 min

Cook time: 30 min

Total time: 35 min

Serving: 6

INGREDIENTS

- 1-pound lean ground beef
- ¼ cup of chopped onion
- ¼ cup of chopped green bell pepper
- ¾ cup of ketchup, or to taste
- 1 tbsp brown sugar, or to taste
- 1 tsp yellow mustard, or to taste
- ½ tsp garlic powder
- salt and ground black pepper to taste
- 6 hamburger buns, split

INSTRUCTIONS

1. Warm up a big skillet in a medium-sized pan. While stirring occasionally, cook lean ground beef in the heated pan for three or four minutes until fat begins to render. After 3–5 minutes, add the onion and bell pepper and simmer until the veggies are tender and the beef is no longer pink in the middle.
2. Add garlic powder, ketchup, brown sugar, mustard, and salt and pepper; stir to combine. Bring to a simmer over low heat for twenty to thirty minutes.
3. Sandwich buns should be uniformly filled with meat mixture.

14. Citrus pork tenderloin

Prep time: 15 min

Cook time: 30 min

Total time: 45 min

Serving: 8

INGREDIENTS

- 2 pork tenderloins
- 2 cloves garlic, sliced or more to taste
- salt and ground black pepper to taste
- 3 blood oranges, halved
- 1 cup of fruity white wine, such as Sauvignon Blanc
- ¼ cup of coarsely chopped cilantro
- 1 tbsp cornstarch
- ½ cup of cold water

INSTRUCTIONS

1. Heat oven to 400 degrees Fahrenheit.
2. Insert a piece of garlic into each tiny, shallow cut made with a sharp paring knife into the pork tenderloins. Before placing the pork in a 9x13-inch glass baking dish, season it with black pepper and salt. Spoon the juice from two or three blood orange halves over the pork before placing it in the oven. Toss the pork with the white wine and garnish with the cilantro.
3. About 30 minutes into baking in a preheated oven, or when a meat thermometer placed into the thickest section of a tenderloin registers 150 degrees Fahrenheit (65 degrees Celsius), check the temperature. After five to ten minutes, set aside the pork to rest.

4. Put the pan juices into a small saucepan and toss out the roasted orange rinds while the pork is resting. Caulk the liquids. Prepare a smooth mixture by whisking cornstarch and cold water in a small basin. Add the mixture to the pan juices. Gently boil sauce for approximately 5 minutes, or until it thickens, with heat reduced to low. Serve with sauce on thinly sliced pork medallions.

15. Asian beef bowls

Prep time: 5 min

Cook time: 10 min

Total time: 15 min

Serving: 4

INGREDIENTS

- ¼ cup of brown sugar, packed
- ¼ cup of reduced-sodium soy sauce
- 2 tsp sesame oil
- ½ tsp crushed red pepper flakes, or more to taste
- ¼ tsp ground ginger
- 1 tbsp vegetable oil
- 3 cloves garlic, minced
- 1 pound ground beef
- 2 green onions, thinly sliced
- ¼ tsp sesame seeds

INSTRUCTIONS

1. Mix well with the brown sugar, ginger, red pepper flakes, sesame oil, soy sauce, and sesame seeds in a small bowl.
2. Warm the vegetable oil in a big cast-iron pan set over medium-high heat. After a minute of continuous stirring, add the garlic and heat until it smells good. Brown the ground beef in a nonstick skillet over medium heat, crumbling it occasionally for three to five minutes. Remove any extra grease.
3. Place the green onions and soy sauce mixture, stir to incorporate, and cook for approximately 2 minutes or until heated.
4. Quickly serve with sesame seeds and green onion, if you like.

16. Bacon and cauliflower casserole

Prep time: 20 min

Cook time: 40 min

Total time: 60 min

Serving: 8

INGREDIENTS

- 3 slices bacon
- 1 head cauliflower (about 2 pounds), cut into bite-size pieces
- ½ tsp ground pepper
- ¼ tsp salt
- 1 ¼ cups of shredded sharp Cheddar cheese, divided
- ⅔ cup of sour cream
- 4 scallions, sliced, divided

INSTRUCTIONS

1. Warm the oven up to 425°F.
2. Cook the bacon for 6 to 8 mins, or until it becomes crisp, in a big nonstick pan set over medium heat. Put on a platter lined with paper towels and set aside to cool. Keep the pan juices aside.
3. In a cooking dish that measures 9 by 13 inches mix the cauliflower,

pepper, salt, and bacon drippings. About 35 minutes into roasting, toss twice to ensure tenderness.

4. In the meantime, mix half of the scallions, 2/3 cup of sour cream, and 1 cup of cheese in a small dish. Incorporate the cheese mixture into the cauliflower while it is still soft. Top with the leftover 1/4 cup of cheese. For a further 5 to 7 minutes, bake until heated.

5. Finely dice the bacon when it has cooled. Bacon and the rest of the scallions should be sprinkled over the heated dish.

17. Cajun beef and rice skillet

Prep time: 10 min

Cook time: 30 min

Total time: 40 min

Serving: 4

INGREDIENTS

- 1-pound lean ground beef (90% lean)
- 3 celery ribs, chopped
- 1 small green pepper, chopped
- 1 small sweet red pepper, chopped
- 1/4 cup of chopped onion
- 2 cups of water
- 1 cup of instant brown rice
- 1 tbsp minced fresh parsley
- 1 tbsp Worcestershire sauce
- 2 tsp reduced-sodium beef bouillon granules
- 1 tsp Cajun seasoning
- 1/4 tsp crushed red pepper flakes
- 1/4 tsp pepper
- 1/8 tsp garlic powder

INSTRUCTIONS

1. After 8 to 10 minutes of cooking in a large pan over medium heat, shred the beef and set aside. Add the celery, green and red peppers, and onion and go on cooking until the meat is no longer pink.

2. Coat the remaining components by stirring them in. Start boiling. Boil gently, cover, and over low heat for 12–15 minutes or until rice reaches desired doneness.

18. Steak Sandwich

Prep time: 20 min

Cook time: 15 min

Total time: 35 min

Serving: 3

INGREDIENTS

- 2 x Red Onion
- 1 x Steak of your choice (Sirloin or Rump work great)
- Rocket
- Sundried Tomatoes
- Rosemary
- Garlic
- Balsamic Vinegar
- Butter
- Extra Virgin Olive Oil
- Red Wine Vinegar
- Olives (optional)

INSTRUCTIONS

1. After chopping an onion thinly, melt a tablespoon of butter in a skillet.

2. Toss in your onions and a bit of salt to the skillet. Reduce heat and

simmer, stirring periodically, for around 15 minutes.

3. Add a few teaspoons of balsamic vinegar after the onions soften, and continue cooking for another 5 minutes or until they are caramelized and extremely delicious.

4. Acquire chopped sundried tomatoes and a handful of fresh rocket greens for the salad. Whisk together the Red Wine Cider Vinegar, Salt, Pepper, and Extra Virgin Olive Oil in a basin. Chopped olives are optionally added.

5. Get a steak—for the best taste, go for rump, ribeye, or sirloin.

6. After that, put it in a skillet and cook it over high heat. Toss it with salt and pepper as per your taste.

7. To get a medium-rare steak, add a small amount of oil to a skillet and sear the steak for two to three minutes on each side.

8. After the steak is cooked, set it aside to rest for a few minutes before slicing it thin.

9. We suggest a crusty, fresh kind of bread for toasting, and then pile on the juicy steak pieces, followed by a heaping amount of balsamic vinegar, caramelized onions, and, last, the rocket salad.

10. Finally, an easy-to-make gourmet steak sandwich right in your kitchen!

19. Easy lamb cutlets

Prep time: 5 min

Cook time: 15 min

Total time: 20 min

Serving: 3

INGREDIENTS

- 5 lamb loin chops
- kosher salt and freshly ground black pepper
- 2 tbsp grass-fed butter — melted. Use ghee if you're doing whole30
- 3 cloves garlic minced
- 1 tsp fresh thyme chopped

INSTRUCTIONS

1. Cook the loin chops 20 to 30 minutes after removing them from the refrigerator. Lay them out on a cutting board lined with paper towels and use them to pat them dry. Add salt and pepper to taste.

2. Turn over medium-high heat and coat a 12-inch cast-iron pan with cooking spray. Put the chops in the pan with the fat side down. You may want to use tongs to hold and press down on the chops to ensure even browning and proper fat rendering. About five minutes.

3. After the fat has melted, place the chops on one side of the pan and press down. Turn and heat for a further three minutes or until browned.

4. Simmer over medium-low heat. Remove the majority of the fat from the lamb using a spoon.

5. Next, combine the garlic, thyme, and 2 tablespoons of butter (or ghee).

6. After the butter has frothed, spoon it over the lamb and let it sit for a minute or two. Toss the lamp chops with the butter sauce and arrange them in a serving dish. Have fun!

20. Ham and brie turnovers

Prep time: 10 min

Cook time: 30 min

Total time: 40 min

Serving: 16

INGREDIENTS

- 1 sheet frozen puff pastry, thawed
- 1/3 cup of apricot preserves
- 4 slices deli ham, quartered
- 8 ounces Brie cheese, cut into 16 pieces

INSTRUCTIONS

1. Turn the oven on high heat (400°). Unroll the puff pastry on a surface gently dusted with flour. Cut the pastry into sixteen 3-inch squares after rolling it out to a 12-inch square. Arrange a spoonful of preserves in the middle of each square. Add ham, bend it if needed, then cheese on top. Place the filling in the center of the pastry, then fold over two opposing corners and squeeze to seal.
2. Line a baking sheet with dish paper and keep aside. Bake for around fifteen to twenty minutes to get a golden-brown color. Let cool for 5 minutes on the pan before you eat. Add more apricot preserves on top if you want.

1. Turkey cabbage soup

Prep time: 1hr

Total time: 1hr

Serving: 4

INGREDIENTS

- 1 lb. Extra Lean Ground Turkey
- 1 Yellow Onion (chopped)
- 3 Garlic (clove, minced)
- 1/2 tsp Dried Thyme
- 2 tbsp Tomato Paste
- 8 cups Chicken Broth
- 2 cups Diced Tomatoes (from the can, with the juice)
- 3 cups Green Cabbage (chopped)
- 3 Carrot (medium, chopped)
- 2 cups Kale Leaves (chopped)
- 2 tbsp Lime Juice
- 1 Red Bell Pepper (diced)
- 1/2 tsp Sea Salt & Black Pepper
- 2 tbsp Parsley (for garnish)

INSTRUCTIONS

1. Toss the chopped onions into a soup pot with the avocado oil and place over medium-low heat. Enough cooking time has passed for the liquid to become transparent.
2. Once the ground turkey stops being pink, add it to the pan. Add the tomato paste, thyme, and garlic, and simmer for one minuter, stirring occasionally.
3. After adding the broth:
4. Whisk in the diced tomatoes.
5. Toss in the carrots and cabbage now.

6. Simmer the covered soup for 10 minutes after bringing it to a low boil.
7. Toss in the bell pepper and kale, then sprinkle with black pepper and sea salt. Keep cooking for another ten minutes. Divide among plates and top with lime juice. When serving, sprinkle with chopped parsley and savor.

2. Speedy chicken cacciatore

Prep time: 3min

Cook time: 12 min

Total time: 15 min

Serving: 3

INGREDIENTS

- 1 tbsp olive oil
- 1 (20-ounce) package of frozen cooked diced chicken breast
- 1 medium-sized green bell pepper, cut into 1-inch pieces
- 1 small onion, cut into 1-inch pieces
- 1 (9-ounce) package of refrigerated angel hair pasta
- 1 (15-ounce) can chunky Italian-style tomato sauce
- 2/3 cup of water
- 1/4 tsp black pepper

INSTRUCTIONS

1. Heat the olive oil in a giant nonstick pan over medium-high heat. When the chicken is browned and the veggies are crisp-tender, add the onion, green pepper, and sauté.
2. Get ready. Add black pepper, tomato sauce, and water to the chicken mixture. Stir to combine. Cook, cover, and over low heat for 5 mins, tossing occasionally. Arrange the spaghetti on four separate dishes. Evenly distribute the chicken mixture over each portion.

3. Chicken Provencal

Prep time: 15 min

Cook time: 1hr

Total time: 1hr 15 min

Serving: 6

INGREDIENTS

- 2 1/2 pounds chicken thighs and legs, bone-in, skin-on
- 2 tbsp Herbs de Provence (store-bought or make your own)
- 10 large garlic cloves, peeled and left whole
- 1 1/2 cups of fresh tomatoes (grape tomatoes, small Roams or cherry tomatoes are nice left whole)
- 1 cup of pitted olives, whole (kalamata or green olives)
- 5 shallots, whole or cut in halves
- 1/2 cup of white wine (sauvignon Blanc is nice)
- 1/2 tsp sea salt, adjust to taste
- 1/2 tsp pepper

INSTRUCTIONS

1. Get the oven to 400 degrees Fahrenheit.
2. Slowly season the chicken with salt and pepper on both sides. Sprinkle the Herbs de Provence generously over the chicken, being sure to press down on all sides.
3. Sear the seasoned chicken for three to five minutes on each side over medium-high heat in a big oven-proof brasier with a cover. Take the pan off the stove.

4. Surround the chicken with the shallots, tomatoes, garlic cloves, and olives. Whisk in the wine and season with pepper and salt. On a cooking sheet covered with foil, roast at 400 grades for 45 minutes to an hour. Ideally, a chicken breast should read 165 degrees Fahrenheit when tested.

4. Wine-poached chicken with herbs and vegetables.

Prep time: 10 min

Cook time: 25 min

Total time: 35 min

Serving: 4

INGREDIENTS

- 2 tsp olive oil
- 1/2 medium onion, chopped
- One and one-half 14.5-ounce cans of whole tomatoes
- 4 skinless chicken breasts
- 1/2 cup of chopped broccoli
- 1/3 cup of chopped red bell pepper
- 1/3 cup of chopped yellow bell pepper
- 1/3 cup of sliced mushrooms
- 2 fresh bay leaves
- 2 sprigs fresh thyme
- Salt and freshly ground black pepper

INSTRUCTIONS

1. Add the oil to an average skillet and sauté the onions over medium heat until they become transparent. Squish the tomatoes in the pan until they become liquid. Simmer the mixture after bringing it to a boil. Chop the red and yellow bell peppers, mushrooms, broccoli, bay leaves, and thyme into the chicken

breasts and stir in. Add salt and pepper to taste. Depending on its thickness, cook the chicken for 8 to 15 minutes or until it's done.

5. Turkey with almond duxelles

Prep time: 10 min

Cook time: 2hr 15 min

Serving: 4

INGREDIENTS

- kg turkey breast, skin off, preferably higher welfare
- sea salt and freshly ground black pepper
- olive oil
- 1 large bunch of fresh thyme leaves picked
- 1 x 340 g jar cranberry jam
- 25 g dried porcini mushrooms
- 6 rashers quality smoked streaky bacon, thinly sliced
- 3 sprigs fresh rosemary
- 600 g mixed mushrooms, chopped
- 1 turkey leg
- 1 carrot, roughly chopped
- 1 leek, trimmed and roughly chopped
- 1 onion, peeled and roughly chopped
- 2 heaped tablespoons plain flour, plus extra for dusting
- 1 tbsp balsamic vinegar
- 1 knob unsalted butter
- 2 x 500 g packets of all butter puff pastry, chilled
- 1 large free-range egg, beaten

INSTRUCTIONS

2. Turn the oven on high heat (180°C/350°F/gas 4). Lay the turkey breast on a board with its breast side down. Delicately cut along the breast muscle's natural connect to create a pocket. Before finishing, add the seasoning and olive oil. After scattering half of the thyme leaves, smooth out the top with cranberry jam and be sure to get into all the crevices. To seal the ingredients inside, fold them back into form in a Swiss-roll manner. To hold it together, press a few cocktail sticks into the seam. Place the turkey on a roasting pan and rub its exterior with the rest of the thyme leaves, a small amount of salt and pepper, and a little olive oil. Coat it evenly, place it in a preheated oven, and roast it for 60 to 70 minutes or until it's almost done (a thermometer should read 72°C at the thickest part).

3. Put the porcini in a bowl of water that has just come to a boil while you wait. To ensure that any grit particles fall to the bottom, stir with a fork after 5 minutes. Fry the bacon in a big skillet with a little oil over average heat for about 5 to 10 minutes or until it becomes a gorgeous golden color and crispy. Add two rosemary sprigs and strip off their leaves during the last 30 seconds. After removing all of the ingredients from the skillet using a slotted spoon, put aside all but the bacon grease. Incorporate the fresh mushrooms into the skillet, along with a dash of pepper and salt. Drain and mince the porcini before adding them to the pan, reserving the water. Before the pan begins to sizzle again and the mushrooms turn golden, soft, sticky, and edged with caramel, add a splash of water, being careful not to include the grit. Cook for approximately 10 to 15 minutes.

4. Slash a small incision into the turkey leg and remove its thigh to create gravy. Combine the leg and thigh with the onion, carrot, and leek in a saucepan. Two liters of boiling water, a decent amount of salt, and flour should be added. Include the balsamic vinegar, the remaining rosemary sprig, and a heaping spoonful of cranberry jam. Return to a boil and simmer, covered, for approximately 2 hours or until thickened. Warm it up before serving after straining it through a sieve.

5. When the pan with the mushrooms has dried up, add a knob of butter and mix to combine. Throw the mushrooms into a food processor and pulse until combined to create a nice blend of smooth and chunky. Allow to cool. You may begin assembling the Wellington when the turkey breast and stuffing cooled.

6. Sprinkle flour on a floured surface. Separate the puff pastry into two equal portions and roll out one to fit a shoe box (one will serve as the foundation, and the other as the lid; make the lid slightly larger than the base). Before adding the smaller pastry sheet, line a large roasting pan with greaseproof paper and sprinkle with flour. Cover an area the size of the turkey breast with half of the mushroom filling spread over the center of the base. After

taking out the cocktail sticks, lay the turkey breast on top. Cover the breast completely by packing and spreading the remaining Filling. Sprinkle with crispy bacon and rosemary after brushing the pastry borders with beaten egg. Carefully form the second layer of pastry to fit the breast shape, pressing out any air bubbles, and then seal it in place. To make the pastry look like the one in the image, trim the edges to about 4 cm. Then, pull, twist, tuck, and pinch to seal.

7. The final step is to brush the entire surface with the beaten egg. Until you're ready to cook it, let it sit uncovered in the fridge overnight. Cook the turkey for 50 to 60 minutes at 180°/350°F/gas 4 on Christmas day, or until it has risen, puffed up, become a gorgeous golden color, and heated through. After taking it out of the oven, let it cool for about 10 minutes before carving. With the gravy and all the customary fixings, serve sliced into 2.5 cm slices. A bite of Christmas.

6. One pan chicken dinner

Prep time: 10 min

Cook time: 1hr

Total time: 1hr 10 min

Serving: 4

INGREDIENTS

- 8 pieces Chicken Breast and or Drumsticks and or Thighs with skin on
- 2 cups of Petite Potatoes
- 2 cups of Baby Carrots
- 1 medium Onion cut to the size of baby carrots
- 1/2 cup of Olive Oil
- 1/2 cup of Salad Dressing We used Brianna's Cilantro Lime
- 2 tsp Montreal Seasoning
- 2 tsp Salt
- 1 tsp Pepper
- 1 tsp Garlic Powder

INSTRUCTIONS

1. On a 12-by-18-inch roasting pan, arrange the chicken, potatoes, carrots, and onions.
2. Combine the spices, oil, and dressing in a bowl.
3. Spread the mixture evenly over the chicken by drizzling it on top and then covering it with a spatula.
4. For a crispier exterior, broil for the last two to three minutes after baking at 400 degrees.

7. Spicy chicken drumsticks

Prep time: 15 min

Cook time: 2hr

Total time: 2hr 15 min

Serving:

INGREDIENTS

- 2 lbs. chicken, skin on, bone-in thighs and legs
- 2 tbsp olive oil
- 2 1/2 teaspoons salt (use 1 teaspoon salt per pound of chicken plus an extra 1/2 teaspoon for the onions)
- 1–2 tsp cracked pepper
- 2 tbsp Lebanese 7-spice

- 1 extra-large red onion, sliced into 1/2-inch wedges
- 4 garlic cloves, roughly chopped
- 1 tbsp preserved lemon, chopped (totally optional)
- 1 lemon, sliced thinly
- 1/4 cup of Marconi almonds, or slivered almonds or peanuts
- parsley for garnish

Seven Spice Recipe:

- 1 tsp cumin
- 1 tsp allspice
- 1 tsp cinnamon
- 1 tsp coriander
- 1/2 tsp ground cloves
- 1/2 tsp nutmeg
- 1/4 tsp cardamom

INSTRUCTIONS

1. Preheat the oven to 400 degrees Fahrenheit.
2. Toss the chicken in a bowl with the 7-spice blend, salt, olive oil, and garlic. Then, stir in the garlic, onion, preserved lemon, and sliced lemon. Preheat a sheet pan and line it with parchment paper.
3. Bake it for 35 to 45 minutes or till done. To get a crisp and golden skin, broil the chicken for a few minutes, flipping it over if needed (particularly important with skin-on chicken).
4. Toss the almonds and pine nuts with olive oil or butter and toast them while the chicken bakes. Add salt and pepper to taste. Remove off the table.
5. Scatter the onions and edible lemon pieces over the aromatic chicken before placing them on a plate. Finish by pouring the pan juices over the top. Add some roasted nuts and chopped parsley for garnish.

8. Thanksgiving turkey breast

Prep time: 15 min

Cook time: 1hr 35 min

Total time: 1hr 50 min

Serving: 4

INGREDIENTS

- ¼ cup of butter softened
- 1 clove garlic, minced
- 1 tsp paprika
- 1 tsp Italian seasoning
- ½ tsp salt-free garlic and herb seasoning blend (such as Mrs. Dash)
- salt and ground black pepper to taste
- 1 (3 pound) turkey breast with skin
- 1 tsp minced shallot
- 1 tbsp butter
- 1 splash of dry white wine
- 1 cup of chicken stock
- 3 tbsp all-purpose flour
- 2 tbsp half-and-half (Optional)

INSTRUCTIONS

1. Get the oven hot, about 350 degrees Fahrenheit (175 degrees Celsius).
2. Toss 1/4 cup of butter, paprika, garlic, Italian spice, garlic and herb seasoning, salt, and black pepper in a bowl.
3. Put the skin-side-up turkey breast in a roasting pan. Gently remove the skin from the turkey breast using your fingers. Then, coat the breast and underside with half of

the butter mixture. Keep the leftover butter mixture aside. Use aluminum foil to tent the turkey breast loosely.

4. Bake the turkey breast for one hour in a preheated oven, and use the leftover butter mixture to baste. Roast for another 30 minutes, or until the pan juices run clear and a meat thermometer put into the thickest part of the breast (without touching the bone) reads 165 degrees Fahrenheit (65 degrees Celsius). Ten to fifteen minutes before serving, allow the turkey breast to rest.

5. Move the pan juices to a skillet while the turkey is resting. Excess fat should be skimmed off, leaving approximately 1 tablespoon in the pan. Set skillet over low heat and sauté shallot in turkey fat, stirring occasionally, until translucent, approximately 5 minutes.

6. Whisk in white wine while melting 1 tablespoon of butter in a saucepan with the shallot; scrape off any browned parts from the pan. Blend in the flour and chicken stock with a whisk. Deduct heat to low and simmer, stirring continuously, until the mixture thickens. Add half-and-half and stir to make a lighter sauce with more creaminess.

7. Enjoy while hot!

9. Chicken Caesar salad

Prep time: 20 min

Cook time: 20 min

Total time: 40 min

Serving: 5

INGREDIENTS
DRESSING

- 1 cup of mayonnaise (Hellman's or S&W Whole Egg) (Note 1)
- 1/2 tsp garlic, finely minced (use a garlic press, if you can)
- 2 anchovy fillets or 3/4 tsp Anchovy paste
- 2 tbsp fresh lemon juice
- 1 tsp Dijon mustard1 tsp Worcestershire sauce
- 1/2 cup of freshly grated parmesan cheese, or 1/3 cup store-bought grated parmesan cheese
- 3 - 4 tbsp milk (to adjust consistency)1/4 tsp salt
- 1/4 tsp Black pepper

GARLIC CROUTONS

- 2 - 3 slices white bread, 2/3" / 1.5cm thick (Note 4)
- 1 garlic, cut in half
- 1 tbsp olive oil
- 1/4 tsp salt

SALAD

- 150g / 5oz streaky bacon, cooked and chopped
- 10 cups cos/romaine lettuce, chopped, washed & dried (1 large, 2 media, 3 small)
- Freshly grated parmesan, for garnish

OPTIONAL EXTRAS - CHICKEN & EGG

- 2 - 4 eggs, cooked to your taste, peeled and halved
- 500g / 1lb chicken breast fillets (2 pieces)
- 1/2 tsp EACH salt and pepper
- 1 tbsp olive oil

INSTRUCTIONS

How to dress

- Puree all the elements in a food processor, beginning with 3 tablespoons of milk.
- Add salt, pepper according to taste, and milk to thin the dressing if needed.
- To let the flavors, develop, set aside for at least 20 minutes.
- BACON
- Put the bacon in a cold skillet and cook it over medium heat without oil. Fry until golden, then flip and cook until golden on the other side. Once cooled, transfer to paper towels and chop.

CROUTOS DE GARLIC

- preheat oven temperature to 180°C (350°F).
- The bread should be toasted for one minute in the toaster or two minutes in the oven on each side or until it is dried out but not browned.
- Spread the sliced side of the garlic over both slices of bread.
- Cut the bread into cubes, about 1.5 cups, and remove the crust if using. After seasoning it with salt and drizzling it with 1–2 tablespoons of olive oil, bake it, shaking the tray

once until brown. It will take around 7 minutes for sandwich bread and 12 to 15 minutes for sourdough and similar loaves.

The assembly processes

- Mix half of the dressing with the lettuce in a bowl. Mix well and add more seasoning if you want.
- Place in a bowl and serve. (Optional: garnish with fried egg and chicken.) On top, sprinkle with croutons and bacon. Before serving, top with parmesan.
- Extras: Chicken and Eggs (Optional)

Laying an Egg:

- Boil some water and add the eggs to a pot.
- Simmer while placed over medium-high heat.
- Simmer the water for 3 minutes if you want soft yolks, 4 minutes if you want firm centers and 6 minutes if you want hard-boiled eggs.
- Take out the eggs, rinse them under cold water for a minute, and then sit in a basin of ice water for five minutes.
- Once peeled, leave aside. For the chicken, you may cut each breast horizontally or pound it until it is approximately 1.2 cm/ 1/2" thick. Add a little salt and pepper on both sides. Put the rendered bacon fat into use. After 5 minutes, flip and cook for 2 more minutes on the other side. After removing, loosely cover it with foil and let it rest for 5 minutes. Slice thinly.

10. Taco stuffed sweet potato.

Prep time: 10 min

Cook time: 20 min

Total time: 30 min

Serving: 4

INGREDIENTS

- 2 sweet potatoes, about 1 pound each
- 1 TBSP avocado oil
- 1-pound lean ground beef
- 1 tbsp chili powder
- 1 tbsp ground cumin
- ½ tsp garlic powder
- ½ tsp onion powder
- ¼ tsp ground chipotle
- ¼ tsp salt
- ¼ cup of water
- 2 tbsp tomato paste
- 1 cup of shredded Mexican cheese blend, divided
- 1 cup of shredded romaine lettuce
- 4 tbsp Pico de Gallo

INSTRUCTIONS

1. prick the sweet potatoes all over. Cook for 10 to 12 mins on High heat or until tender.
2. Set aside a big skillet over medium-high heat to heat the oil. Spice up your beef with chili powder, cumin, garlic powder, onion powder, chipotle, and salt. Brown the meat, and tear it up with a wooden spoon until it's no longer pink, which should take around 4 to 6 minutes. In a measuring cup, whisk together the tomato paste and water. Transfer the mixture to the pan and swirl to combine. Coat with half a cup of cheese.
3. Cut the sweet potatoes in half and use a fork to mash the flesh. Divide the beef mixture in half and top with half a cup, followed by two tablespoons of cheese, a quarter cup of lettuce, and one tablespoon of Pico de Gallo.

11. Rosemary chicken with potatoes and beans

Prep time: 15 min

Cook time: 30 min

Total time: 45 min

Serving: 4

INGREDIENTS

- 6 (about 1 pound) small red potatoes (2"), cut into fourths
- 1 cup of chicken broth
- 2 TBSP butter
- 3-4 (24 ounces) Gold's Plump® Boneless Skinless Chicken Breasts
- 2 cups of cut fresh green beans (2 inches in length)
- 1 tsp dried rosemary
- 1/4 tsp pepper

INSTRUCTIONS

1. Add the potatoes and half a cup of chicken stock in a big nonstick pan. Raise the heat to high and get a boil. Wrap and cook on low heat for 10 minutes to get the potatoes almost soft. Take the potatoes out of the pan and put them aside.
2. While the pan is hot, melt the butter. When the chicken is just beginning to brown, add to the pan and cook, stirring once, for 6

minutes. Toss the chicken with the green beans, half a cup of chicken stock, rosemary, pepper, and potatoes that are half cooked.

3. Raise the heat to high and get a boil. Simmer, covered, for 10 minutes or until beans and potatoes are soft and chicken reaches an internal temperature of 170°F.

4. Add green beans, potatoes, and pan juices to the chicken dish.

12. Chicken with lemon caper pan sauces

Prep time: 10 min

Cook time: 35 min

Total time: 45 min

Serving: 4

INGREDIENTS

- 2 8-ounce boneless, skinless chicken breasts
- ½ tsp salt, divided
- ½ tsp ground pepper, divided
- ¼ cup of white whole-wheat flour
- 3 tbsp extra-virgin olive oil, divided
- ½ cup of thinly sliced leek
- 2 tbsp sliced shallot
- 1 tbsp lemon zest
- ¼ cup of lemon juice
- 1 cup of low-sodium chicken broth
- 1 tbsp capers
- 1 tbsp butter

INSTRUCTIONS

1. If the chicken tenders are still connected, remove them and set aside. Cut the breasts in half lengthwise; you should end up with four equal pieces. Spread out on a chopping board and wrap in a big plastic bag. Flatten to a thickness of approximately 1/4 inch by pounding with the smooth side of a meat mallet or a heavy saucepan. Put 1/4 tsp of pepper and 1/4 teaspoon of salt. Coat the cutlets in flour, being sure to shake off any excess, and set them aside in a shallow dish. (Spill the rest of the flour.)

2. A giant skillet over medium-high heat should be heated with 2 teaspoons of oil. Cook the chicken for 2–3 minutes on each side or until browned and cooked, flipping once. Cover with foil and transfer to a large serving platter to maintain warmth. Carry out the same process with the reserved chicken.

3. Put the shallot, leek, and the remaining tablespoon of oil in the pan. Just till tender, about 1 to 2 minutes, while stirring occasionally in the pan. get boil and add the lemon juice. Reduce the lemon juice by half, approximately 45 seconds, while scraping out any browned pieces from the pan's bottom. Toss with pepper and 1/4 tsp of salt. Stir in the broth, zest, and capers. For approximately 4–7 minutes, while stirring occasionally, reduce the sauce by half. Take it off the stove and mix in the butter. Place the sauce over the chicken and serve.

13. Italian chicken thighs

Prep time: 10 min

Cook time: 45 min

Total time: 55 min

Serving: 2

INGREDIENTS

- 1 lb. chicken thighs bone-in
- 1 tbsp garlic powder
- 1 tsp red pepper flakes
- 1 tsp dried oregano
- 1 tsp sea salt

INSTRUCTIONS

1. Preheat and Cook in an oven heated to 425°F. Use cooking paper to line a baking sheet.
2. In a small bowl, combine the red pepper flakes, oregano, salt, garlic powder, and red pepper.
3. After patting the chicken thighs dry, set it on a baking sheet.
4. Season with half the seasonings, half on each side.
5. Cook the thighs in the oven for around 45 minutes or until fully done.

14. Spicy cacciatore

Prep time: 5 min

Cook time: 1hr 15 min

Total time: 1hr 20 min

Serving: 4

INGREDIENTS

- 1 tbsp olive oil
- 4 chicken leg portions, skin on
- 2 red peppers, deseeded and cut into strips
- 1 medium red chili, deseeded and sliced
- glass red wine (about 175ml/6fl oz)
- ½ quantity tomato sauce (see 'Goes well with')
- 1-2 handfuls black olives
- chopped flatleaf parsley to serve

INSTRUCTIONS

1. Bake at 180 degrees Celsius (160 degrees fan) using gas 4. Heat the oil in a deep, ovenproof roasting pan large enough to accommodate the chicken in one layer. After seasoning the chicken pieces evenly, put the pan on the stove and brown them for 7 to 10 minutes per side over medium heat. Use a spoon to remove the chicken and set it aside.
2. Sauté the peppers and chili in the remaining grease for about 10 minutes or until they are soft and starting to brown on the edges. After removing any extra fat, add the wine and swirl thoroughly for one or two minutes until it bubbles up. Add the tomato sauce and stir one more. To get a thick pouring consistency, add a small amount of water (up to 150ml) after you've tossed the chicken in the sauce, and top with olives. To get a crispy chicken, cover and bake for 30 minutes. After that, uncover and cook for another 15-20 minutes. Remove any excess fat by spooning it off, topping it with chopped parsley, and serving it over mashed potatoes, polenta, or rice.

15. Chicken wings with parmesan sauce

Prep time: 10 min

Cook time: 35 min

Total time: 45 min

Serving: 4

INGREDIENTS

- 1.5 lbs. chicken wings (10 pieces)

- 1 tsp garlic powder
- 1/2 tsp dried oregano
- 1/4 tsp salt + more for the water
- 1/2 cup of freshly grated Parmesan cheese
- 1/4 cup of unsalted butter melted

INSTRUCTIONS

1. Set oven temperature to 450 degrees Fahrenheit.
2. Bring a large saucepan of water to a boil. Just like you would while making pasta, season the water with salt. The water should have a somewhat repulsive saltiness, like seawater if you taste it.
3. After 7 or 8 minutes in the boiling water, remove the wings from the pot and pat them dry using a paper towel. They won't bake up crispy unless you pat them dry first.
4. Spread the wings out on a cooking sheet, fat side down. Bake for 25 to 30 minutes till hash browns. Turn the wings over and bake for 5 more minutes. On the side that touched the pan, the skin should appear crackly golden and crispy.
5. Toss the chicken pieces in a combination of garlic powder, oregano, salt, Parmesan, and butter. I hope you savor it!

16. Chicken fajitas

Prep time: 10 min

Cook time: 25 min

Total time: 35 min

Serving: 4

INGREDIENTS
FOR THE FAJITA SEASONING:

- 2 tsp. Onion Powder
- 1 tsp. Garlic Powder
- 1 tsp. Cumin
- 1/2 tsp. Oregano
- 1/2 tsp. Paprika
- 1/2 tsp. Black Pepper
- 3/4 tsp. Salt

FOR THE CHICKEN AND VEGETABLES:

- 2 Large Boneless, Skinless Chicken Breasts
- 1 Medium Red Onion, Thinly Sliced
- 1 Red Bell Pepper, Sliced
- 1 Green Bell Pepper, Sliced
- Tortillas, Sour Cream, Avocado, Cilantro, And Lime For Serving (optional)

INSTRUCTIONS

1. To make the fajita seasoning, combine all ingredients in a small bowl and whisk.
2. If you're making chicken and veggies:
3. Warm the oven up to 425°F.
4. Rub fajita spice on both the inside and outside of the chicken breasts. Remove off the table.
5. On a rimmed baking sheet, distribute the peppers and onion equally. Top with the seasoned chicken. About 22-30 minutes into the baking time, check that the internal heat of the chicken reaches 165°F in the thickest area. Let the chicken sit for 10 minutes after transferring it to a platter. While the chicken is resting, bake the vegetables for a little longer if they aren't done to your taste.
6. With the vegetables, slice the chicken and serve. Additional

toppings include tortillas, sour cream, avocado, cilantro, and lime juice.

17. Chicken shawarma

Prep time: 10 min

Cook time: 15 min

Marinating time: 6hr

Serving: 4

INGREDIENTS

- 2 lbs. chicken thighs boneless, skinless
- 2 tsp kosher salt
- 1 tbsp garlic paste
- 2 tsp paprika
- ½ tsp cayenne pepper
- 1 tsp ground cumin
- 1 tsp ground coriander
- ½ tsp ground cinnamon
- ½ tsp ground cardamom
- ½ tsp ground cloves
- ½ tsp ground black pepper
- 2 tbsp lemon juice
- 2 tbsp oil

Dill Tzatziki sauce

- 1 cup of Greek-style plain yogurt
- 2 Persian cucumbers peeled and grated (squeeze excess moisture out)
- 1 clove garlic minced
- 1 tbsp lemon juice freshly squeezed
- 2 tbsp fresh dill finely chopped
- ½ tsp kosher salt
- ¼ tsp freshly ground black pepper
- Serving
- pita bread or parathas
- 2 cups of Romaine lettuce
- 2 tomatoes diced

- 2 Persian cucumbers peeled and cubed
- ½ cup of red onion thinly sliced

INSTRUCTIONS

- Combine the following ingredients in a big basin: salt, garlic, paprika, cayenne pepper, black pepper, cumin, coriander, cinnamon, cardamom, cloves, oil, and ground cumin.
- Dredge the chicken in the mixture. Half an hour or more is plenty of time to marinate.
- Gather all the necessary ingredients and set the air fryer to 400 degrees Fahrenheit. Separate the chicken breasts into one layer. Before serving, top with sliced onions. Bake in an air fryer at 380 degrees Fahrenheit for 10 minutes. Cook for more 2 to 5 minutes after turning. Just a heads up: you can put four or five chicken thighs into my air fryer basket without any problems. Air frying chicken requires two batches for me.
- After 2 minutes of resting, slice the chicken into thin strips.

Pita bread

- Combine the mango, cucumber, garlic, lemon juice, and dill with the yoghurt in a medium bowl. Add salt and pepper to taste.

Bread

- Get the pita, flatbread, or paratha breads warm.
- Serving
- The traditional method to eat shawarma is with tzatziki spread on warm bread. Then, pile on your

preferred vegetables: tomato and lettuce. Afterwards, arrange the chicken slices on top. Rise and savor.

- Make them into pita pockets if you choose. Turn the toaster oven high and cook the pita bread until it puffs up. Once it has cooled for a minute, slice it in half. Carefully split the pita bread in half and stuff with tzatziki. Pile on the tomatoes, lettuce, and chicken.

- Shawarma meat, a bed of crunchy lettuce, tomatoes, and cucumbers, and a dollop of creamy yoghurt Tzatziki make for a low-carb dinner.

18. Turkey schnitzel

Prep time: 10 min

Cook time: 20 min

Total time: 30 min

Serving: 4

INGREDIENTS

- 1/4 cup of 2% milk
- 1/2 cup of all-purpose flour
- 2 eggs, lightly beaten
- 3/4 cup of seasoned bread crumbs
- 1 pound turkey slices (1/4 inch thick)
- 2 tbsp butter
- 2 tbsp canola oil

INSTRUCTIONS

1. Combine the milk, flour, eggs, and breadcrumbs in four individual little basins. Before coating it with flour, dip the turkey pieces in milk. Roll in bread crumbs and then into eggs.

Lay out on waxed paper and allow to rest for 5 to 10 minutes.

2. Sauté the turkey in a big pan with the oil and butter over average-high heat for 2 minutes per side or until the juices drain away.

19. Chicken quesadillas

Prep time: 5 min

Cook time: 15 min

Total time: 20 min

Serving: 2

INGREDIENTS

- 500 grams of chicken strips
- 1 tsp cumin
- 4 garlic cloves, minced
- 1 bunch coriander
- 1 pack Tortillas
- 500 grams of Sermon Mozzarella, grated
- 1 large red onion, sliced
- 4 habanero chilies, chopped

INSTRUCTIONS

1. Cook the chicken, garlic, and cumin in a pan with oil over medium heat for 5 minutes. Before adding the red onion, turn off the heat and let it simmer for another 5 minutes.

2. Place one tortilla on a plate and top it with the chicken, mozzarella, cilantro, and habanero peppers. Before serving, place the second tortilla on top. Apply a generous thin layer of oil on the tortilla.

3. Place the filled tortilla, oil side down, in a large nonstick skillet and cook for three minutes until lightly browned. After a cautious turn, cook for 2 minutes or until golden. Cut into wedges before serving.

20. Chicken lettuce wraps

Prep time: 20 min

Cook time: 20 min

Total time: 40 min

Serving: 2-4

INGREDIENTS

- 3 to 5 tbsp hoisin sauce (gluten-free, if needed)
- 2 tbsp soy sauce (or 1 tablespoon tamari or coconut aminos if gluten-free)
- 2 tbsp rice vinegar
- 1 tsp toasted sesame oil
- 1 tsp cornstarch (optional)
- 1 pound ground chicken or ground turkey
- 2 tsp vegetable oil, divided
- 8 ounces white button or cremini mushrooms, finely chopped
- Optional vegetables: finely diced onions, diced bell peppers, finely diced or grated carrots
- 1 (8-ounce) can water chestnuts, drained and finely chopped
- 3 cloves garlic, minced
- 1 tbsp peeled and minced fresh ginger
- 1/2 cup thinly sliced scallions (from about 6 scallions), divided
- 2 small heads of Bibb or butter lettuce
- Serving options: red pepper flakes, hot sauce

INSTRUCTIONS

1. Prepare the sauce. Mix the hoisin sauce, soy sauce, rice vinegar, and sesame oil; add 3 tablespoons of each. Whisk in the cornstarch for a thicker, glossier sauce; set aside and keep close to the heat.
2. First, brown the ground chicken. To make the oil shimmer:
3. Heat 1 teaspoon in a big skillet over medium heat.
4. Cook, stirring slowly, for 7 to 8 minutes or until the ground chicken is no longer pink and cooked through.
5. Move the cooked chicken to a separate, clean bowl and put it aside.
6. Bring the aromatics and veggies to a boil. Transfer the remaining 1 teaspoon of oil to the same skillet. After about four or five minutes of cooking, add the mushrooms and any extra veggies you'd like. Stir occasionally to prevent them from sticking. When the water chestnuts, garlic, and ginger are fragrant, which should take approximately 30 seconds, stir them in.
7. Add the chicken and veggies and mix well. Put half of the scallions in the pan and add the chicken back.
8. Toss the sauce in. Cook, stirring regularly, for 30 to 60 seconds or until the sauce is heated through and bubbling. If you want it to be spicy, add extra hoisin sauce.
9. Top with lettuce and serve. Place a heap of lettuce leaves on a plate in the middle of the table. Arrange on top of the lettuce in tiny dishes, and place the spicy sauce, red pepper flakes, and chopped scallions. Serve and transfer to a serving platter when heated. Spoon some chicken mixture into the center of each lettuce leaf, garnish with scallions and spicy sauce or red pepper flakes, and serve immediately. Each person can have a spoon.

1. Fresh dill dip

Prep time: 15 min

Total time: 15 min

Serving: 6

INGREDIENTS:

- 1 Cup of sour cream
- 1 Cup of mayonnaise
- 1/2 tsp onion powder
- 1/2 tbsp garlic powder
- 4 1/2 tbsp of fresh dill, finely chopped
- 1 tbsp of fresh parsley, finely chopped

INSTRUCTIONS

1. In a bowl, add all the ingredients and stir until well blended. Put in the fridge for at least an hour before serving with chips, crackers, or vegetables.

2. Instant popcorn

Prep time: 5 min

Cook time: 18 min

Total time: 23 min

Serving: 4

INGREDIENTS

- 3 tbsp clarified butter ghee or coconut oil
- ¾ cup of popcorn kernels
- 2 tsp salt

INSTRUCTIONS

2. Arrange all the ingredients in a row close to the stove. Put the wooden spatula and glass lid by the pot.
3. Once the light is on MORE, choose SAUTE and tweak it as needed. Hold on until the temperature gauge reads HOT.
4. While it's melting, stir in some clarified butter or coconut oil. You should hold off until you hear the sizzling of oil.
5. Toss in some salt. Lift the inner pot and swirl it around to coat the base with oil and salt, using two kitchen towels to keep your hand from burning.
6. Put some popcorn kernels in the saucepan and wait for them to pop. It may be a moment before these finishes. Once the kernels of popcorn are heated, they will pop.
7. Add the remaining popcorn kernels after you hear a few pops. Place the glass cover on top to allow steam to escape, leaving a small gap.
8. After about 30 seconds, lift the inner pot and shake it.
9. It will take around three or four minutes for the popcorn to pop. There will be more popping.
10. When the popping stops, or when you can count to three, take the inner pot out of the heat and set it aside for a minute or two to cool. Any kernels that haven't been popped will eventually pop. The goal is to pop "almost" every kernel of popcorn.
11. Gently agitate the pop one more. Serve immediately in serving popcorn tubs and season to taste as described before.

3. Radish chip

Prep time: 10 min

Cook time: 10 min

Total time: 20 min

Serving: 4

INGREDIENTS

- Oil for deep frying, preferably palm oil
- 16 oz radishes
- 1/2 tsp coarse salt, kosher or sea

INSTRUCTIONS

1. A heavy saucepan or deep-fat fryer should be heated to 325 degrees Fahrenheit with 2 to 3 inches of oil.
2. Radishes should be thinly sliced using a mandolin or sharp knife.
3. Add water to a saucepan and add the radishes. Heat until it boils. After 4–5 minutes of boiling, the radishes should be transparent, and the skins should brighten. Use a colander to drain the radish slices.
4. To avoid splattering, carefully add the sliced radishes to the heated oil.
5. For a rich golden-brown color, fry radish slices in heated oil for 8 to 10 minutes.
6. Before seasoning, drain on paper towels.

4. Quinoa and white bean loaf

Prep time: 20 min

Cook time: 20 min

Total time: 40 min

Serving: 2

INGREDIENTS

Stew

- 1 tbsp olive oil
- ½ medium red onion, diced
- ½ cup of quinoa, rinsed and drained
- 1 cup of shredded carrots
- 1 to 2 cups vegetable broth
- 2 cups of canned tomatoes, drained
- ½ tsp sea salt
- ½ tsp black pepper
- 1 cup of canned cannellini beans
- Parsley Pesto
- 1 clove garlic
- 1 cup of parsley
- 2 tbsp olive oil
- 2 tbsp lemon juice
- 1 tbsp toasted pine nuts, plus more to garnish

INSTRUCTIONS

1. One tbsp of olive oil should be heated in a large saucepan over medium heat. Proceed to sauté the onions for another 4 to 5 minutes or until they become tender. Toss in the quinoa, carrots, tomato puree, 1 cup of broth, ground pepper, and salt. After bringing it to a boil, simmer it for 12–15 minutes or until the quinoa is soft. Cook for a further 5 minutes after stirring in the cannellini beans. Add vegetable

broth if the stew has thickened excessively to get the correct consistency.

2. In a food processor, pulse the garlic while the stew is cooking. Parsley, olive oil, lemon juice, and pine nuts should be added. If necessary, thin it with 1–2 tablespoons of water and pulse until thoroughly blended.

3. Incorporate the pesto into the broth after scooping it into two plates. Toast the bread and sprinkle with more pine nuts before serving. This stew may be prepared in advance. Reheat it gently, adding more broth if necessary.

5. Roasted veggies bowl

Prep time: 10 min

Cook time: 50 min

Total time: 1hr

Serving: 4

INGREDIENTS

FARRO

- 1 ½ cups of farro (300 g), soaked for 30 min
- 3 cups of water (720 mL)

ROASTED VEGGIES

- 3 cups of Private Selection Petite Medley Potatoes (675 g)
- 1 cup of carrot (120 g), sliced
- olive oil, to taste
- garlic powder, to taste
- kosher salt, to taste
- pepper, to taste
- 1 cup of broccoli floret (150 g)

MARINATED TOFU

- 2 tbsp olive oil
- ½ tsp dried thyme
- ½ tsp dried oregano
- 1 clove garlic, grated
- kosher salt, to taste
- pepper, to taste
- 1 cup of extra firm tofu (250 g), pressed and cubed

ROASTED CHICKPEAS

- 1 cup of canned chickpea (200 g), drained and rinsed
- olive oil, to taste
- kosher salt, to taste
- ¼ tsp paprika
- ¼ tsp chili powder

LEMON TAHINI DRESSING

- ½ cup of tahini (120 mL)
- ¼ cup of water (60 mL)
- 1 tbsp olive oil
- 1 tbsp lemon juice
- ¼ tsp kosher salt

INGREDIENTS

- Have you got your oven preheated to 375°F or 190 °C?
- The farro may be prepared by bringing a medium saucepan of water and farro to a boil over high heat. After 20–25 minutes of simmering, covered, over low heat, the farro should be soft and the water absorbed.

Get the vegetables ready to roast:

- Halve the potatoes.
- Place half the vegetables on one baking sheet and the carrots on the other.

- Toss with olive oil and add salt, pepper, and garlic powder.
- Coat thoroughly by tossing.
- Give it a quick bake for 10 minutes.
- After taking it out of the oven, put the broccoli on the baking sheet. Olive oil, salt, garlic powder, and pepper should be sprinkled over top. Go on cooking for another 15 to 20 minutes or until vegetables are soft to the touch.
- To prepare the marinated tofu:
- Mix the olive oil, garlic, thyme, oregano, salt, and pepper in a small dish.
- Coat the tofu by adding it and stirring.
- Reserve for a further ten minutes.
- Place the tofu on a half-full baking pan. Take it out of the oven and give it a quick turn after 20 minutes.

To roast the chickpeas,

- Lay them on top of the tofu on the other side of the oven pan.
- After seasoning it with salt, paprika, and chili powder, drizzle it with olive oil.
- Oat thoroughly by tossing.
- The chickpeas should be crunchy after another fifteen minutes in the oven.
- To make the lemon tahini dressing, first, kick the tahini with water, olive oil, lemon juice, and salt in a liquid measuring cup till thoroughly blended.
- Arrange the roasted vegetables, tofu, and chickpeas on top of the farro to make the grain bowl. Spread the tahini sauce on top.

- Have fun!

6. Veggies fajitas

Prep time: 10 min

Cook time: 15 min

Total time: 25 min

Serving: 6

INGREDIENTS

- 3 tbsp olive oil
- 3 bell peppers - seeds and stems removed, sliced into thin strips
- 1 red onion - skin and ends removed, sliced into half-moons
- ½ tsp dried oregano
- ½ tsp ground cumin
- ¼ tsp salt - more to taste

INSTRUCTIONS

1. Warm the olive oil in a pan set over average-high heat until it becomes hot and aromatic. Toss in the onions and peppers, then top with cumin, salt, oregano, and mix. Although the pan will initially be somewhat full, the vegetables will gradually reduce in size as they cook.
2. Stirring regularly with a wooden spoon, scrape off any brown pieces from the bottom of the skillet, and cook till the vegetables are soft and slightly browned. Continue cooking for about 7 minutes if you want tougher vegetables. It takes ten to fifteen minutes (or more) to have vegetables tender and browned. Add additional salt if needed.
3. Take it off the stove and use it on burritos, tacos, or fajitas.

7. Roasted asparagus

Prep time: 10 min

Cook time: 15 min

Total time: 20 min

Serving: 4

INGREDIENTS

- 1 bunch thin asparagus spears, trimmed
- 3 tbsp olive oil
- 1 ½ tbsp grated Parmesan cheese (Optional)
- 1 clove garlic, minced (Optional)
- 1 tsp sea salt
- ½ tsp ground black pepper
- 1 tbsp lemon juice (Optional)

INSTRUCTION

1. Get the oven hot, about 425 degrees Fahrenheit (220 degrees Celsius).
2. Add the asparagus to a bowl and coat it with olive oil. Toss with salt and pepper, Garlic powder, and Parmesan cheese. Put the asparagus spears on a baking dish in a single layer.
3. Preheat oven to 400 degrees Fahrenheit. Bake for 12–15 minutes, or until almost done.

8. Butternut squash soup

Prep time: 20 min

Cook time: 45 min

Total time: 1hr 5 min

Serving: 4

INGREDIENTS

- 2 tbsp butter
- 1 small onion, chopped
- 1 stalk celery, chopped
- 1 medium carrot, chopped
- 2 medium potatoes, cubed
- 1 medium butternut squash - peeled, seeded, and cubed
- 1 (32 fluid ounces) container of chicken stock
- salt and freshly ground black pepper to taste

INSTRUCTIONS

1. Assemble all of the components.
2. In a giant saucepan, melt the butter over medium heat. Sauté the onion, celery, carrot, potatoes, and squash for approximately 5 minutes or until gently browned. Toss in just enough chicken broth to coat the veggies.
3. Heat until it boils, then deduct heat to medium-high. Simmer and cover over low heat for 40 minutes or until veggies are soft.
4. Blend the soup until it's completely smooth. Return to the saucepan and stir in any leftover stock to get the appropriate consistency. Add salt and pepper to taste.
5. Enjoy while hot!

9. Cauliflower tots

Prep time: 10 min

Cook time: 25 min

Total time: 35 min

Serving: 10

INGREDIENTS

- 550g (1 small head) Cauliflower, cut into cauliflower florets

- 220g (2 small) Carrots, chopped roughly into 1½-2cm (½-1inch) pieces
- ½ Red Bell Pepper (capsicum), finely chopped
- 2 Spring onions (salad / green onion), finely chopped
- 2 tbsp Flat Leaf parsley, finely chopped
- 75g / ¾ Cup of Cheddar Cheese, grated
- 20g / ¼ Cup of Parmesan Cheese
- 2 Eggs, beaten
- 60g / 1 Cup of Panko Breadcrumbs

INSTRUCTIONS

1. Preheat oven temperature to 190°C (375°F). Line a baking sheet with parchment paper.
2. Sauté the carrots for three minutes. Toss in the cauliflower and continue steaming for another 5 to 9 minutes. (Until fork tender)
3. After the carrots and cauliflower are drained, rinse them with cold water. Rinse well and then put in a blender. Be careful not to over-pulse the food processor until the pepper and spring onion are finely minced.
4. Toss the cauliflower mixture with the rest of the ingredients in a large bowl. Combine by gently stirring.
5. Roll out a spoonful of the ingredients into a tot form with your palm. Keep going until you've used up all the mixture. There should be about 33 toddlers.
6. Spray with oil (optional) and place on the baking sheet; bake for 20 - 25 minutes.

10. Garlic herb sweet potato fries

Prep time: 10 min

Cook time: 30 min

Total time: 40 min

Serving: 4

INGREDIENTS

- 3 sweet potatoes, peeled and sliced into thin, even strips
- 2 tbsp olive oil
- 2 tbsp cornstarch
- 1 tsp onion powder
- 1/2 salt
- 1/4 tsp pepper
- 1/4 tsp dried thyme
- 1/8 tsp red pepper flakes
- 3 cloves garlic, minced
- 2 tbsp fresh parsley, chopped
- 3 tbsp grated parmesan chee

INSTRUCTIONS

1. Heat oven to 400 degrees. Use cooking paper or a baking mat to line a baking sheet.
2. Combine cornstarch, onion powder, onions, pepper, dried thyme, and red pepper flakes in a small bowl and whisk to combine.
3. Combine the sliced sweet potatoes and olive oil in a big basin and mix to combine. Add the cornstarch mixture and whisk. Once the baking sheet is ready, spread the mixture evenly over it.
4. To get a brown color, bake for 20 to 30 minutes. (The thickness of the fries you slice will determine how long it takes.) After taking it out of

the oven, stir in the parsley, garlic, and parmesan cheese.

5. Instantaneous service is required.

11. Zucchini fritter

Prep time: 20 min

Cook time: 25 min

Total time: 45 min

Serving: 4

INGREDIENTS

- 1 ½ pounds zucchini, grated
- ¾ tsp salt
- ¼ cup of all-purpose flour
- ¼ cup of grated Parmesan cheese
- 1 large egg, beaten
- 2 cloves garlic, minced
- kosher salt and ground black pepper to taste
- 2 tbsp olive oil

INSTRUCTIONS

1. In a large colander, combine the zucchini and salt. Set aside to drain for 10 minutes.
2. After transferring the zucchini to the middle of a cheesecloth, wrap it around it and press to extract as much liquid as possible.
3. Toss the garlic, egg, flour, and Parmesan cheese in a large basin. Add the zucchini and stir to combine. Add the kosher salt and pepper.
4. Olive oil must be heated in a big pan over medium-high heat.
5. Drop heaping tbsp of the zucchini mixture into the heated pan in batches and cook, turning once,

until golden brown, approximately 2 minutes on each side.

6. Enjoy while hot!

12. Onion rings

Prep time: 15 min

Cook time: 5 min

Total time: 20 min

Serving: 4

INGREDIENTS

- 1 large sweet or yellow onion, sliced into ½-inch thick rings
- 1 cup of buttermilk
- 1 large egg
- ½ cup of all-purpose flour
- 1 tbsp cornstarch
- 1 tsp smoked paprika
- 1 tsp salt
- ½ tsp black pepper
- ½ tsp garlic powder
- 1 cup of panko bread crumbs
- Oil for frying (canola oil, vegetable oil, or peanut oil are our top choices)

INSTRUCTIONS

1. In a tiny bowl, whisk the egg and buttermilk together.
2. Whisk together the cornstarch, flour, smoked paprika, salt, pepper, and garlic powder in a tiny bowl. Crumbs should be added to a third shallow dish.
3. Before dredging in the buttermilk mixture:
4. Toss the onion rings with the flour mixture.
5. Coat them with breadcrumbs.
6. Wait 10–15 minutes before frying.
7. Coatings tend to break off when fried, but if you let them sit for a

little, they can soak up some moisture and become sticky.

8. In a giant Dutch oven or other heavy-duty pot, heat 1" of oil to a temperature of 350°F to 375°F. Use a cast-iron pan if you like.

9. Fry three or four onion rings at once for two or three minutes on each side, being careful not to overcrowd the pan. Flip the rings halfway through cooking until they are crispy and lightly browned. Place a wire rack over a cooking sheet to remove excess oil and transfer the fried onion rings. Continue with the rest of the rings.

13. Stuffed bell peppers

Prep time: 15 min

Cook time: 50 min

Total time: 1hr 5 min

Serving: 6

INGREDIENTS

- 3 bell peppers
- 2 Tbsp cooking oil, divided
- 1 lb. Italian sausage
- 1 yellow onion, diced
- 3 garlic cloves, minced
- 1 tsp Italian seasoning
- 1/2 tsp garlic powder
- 1 1/4 tsp salt, divided
- 1/4 tsp freshly cracked black pepper
- 1 cup of marinara sauce
- 1/2 cup of uncooked long-grain white rice
- 3/4 cup of chicken broth
- 1 cup of shredded mozzarella

INSTRUCTIONS

1. Turn the oven on high heat (350°F). After you give each bell pepper a good wash and pat dry, slice them horizontally in half. Always aim for an equal cut while cutting them. Carefully cut the top half of each bell pepper off at the stem (see photo below) using a sharp paring knife. A little hole at the stem removal site is just OK.

2. In a casserole dish that measures 9×13 inches, lay each half of the bell pepper. After brushing the bell peppers with 1 tablespoon of oil, add ½ teaspoon of salt and ½ teaspoon of cracked black pepper. Bell peppers may be softened by baking them in a preheated oven for 20 minutes. Set aside the bell peppers after 20 minutes of baking.

3. Prepare the filling ingredients as the bell peppers bake. One tablespoon of oil has been heated in a large pan over medium heat. Get the Italian sausage browned.

4. After the sausage is cooked, add the chopped onion and minced garlic. Once the garlic smells aromatic and the onion softens, sauté for a few more minutes over medium heat.

5. After that, throw in the chicken stock, marinara sauce, garlic powder, 1 tsp of salt, and uncooked rice. Season with Italian seasoning and stir in. Mix thoroughly.

6. Bring the ingredients to a full boil in a covered pan over medium-high heat. Lower the heat to medium-low as soon as it boils and simmer, covered, for 20 minutes. Do not stir. Take out from heat and allow it to rest, covered, for another 5 minutes after 20 minutes.

7. The next step is to take the lid off, give the rice a little fluffing, and toss the mixture one more to give everything a good stir. Put some beef filling into each bell pepper and start stuffing them. Fill each to the brim with as much Filling as you can manage.

8. Distribute the shredded mozzarella cheese equally over the bell peppers. Bake for 15 minutes with a loosely tented aluminum foil over the casserole dish. The peppers should be softened, but not mushy, after 15 minutes.

9. Take the foil off and set the broiler to high. Cook the filled bell peppers under the broiler for two to three minutes or until the cheese begins to color slightly. Keep a tight eye on the bell peppers at this stage to avoid the cheese from browning too much. Finish with a sprinkle of parsley, if you want, and savor!

14. Kale Chips

Prep time: 5min

Cook time: 15 min

Total time: 20 min

Serving: 4

INGREDIENTS

- 6 cups of kale, ribs and stems removed, coarsely chopped
- 1 tbsp Land O Lakes® Butter, melted
- Salt, if desired

INSTRUCTIONS

1. Preheat the oven to 325F. Before you begin, line a cooking sheet with parchment paper.

2. Fill a bowl with kale. Pour in the melted butter and mix until covered well.

3. Lay out the kale on the baking sheet lined with parchment paper. Season with salt to taste.

4. Cook the chips for 14 to 16 minutes or until they are as crisp as you like. Instantaneous service is required.

15. Cold sesame cucumber noodle salad

Prep time: 10 min

Cook time: 30 min

Total time: 40 min

Serving: 4

INGREDIENTS

- 1 lb. thin spaghetti
- 1/2 cup of light sweet miso
- 4 tsp. toasted sesame oil
- 4 tsp. light brown sugar
- 2 fresh limes, juiced
- 1 garlic clove, minced
- 1/3 cup of grapeseed oil
- 1 red bell pepper, small diced
- 2 small cucumbers, sliced
- 4 green onions, chopped

For serving (optional):

- Sesame seeds
- Fresh limes, sliced
- Green onions, chopped

INSTRUCTIONS

- In a giant pot, boil water for pasta. Add spaghetti and stir to prevent sticking. Cook according to package instructions.

- Whisk miso, sesame oil, brown sugar, lime juice, and garlic in a large bowl. Slowly stream in oil as you whisk until the sauce is smooth and thick. Whisk in 2 tablespoons water.
- Drain spaghetti and rinse with cold water. Shake off any excess water and add to bowl with sauce. Toss to coat evenly. Add bell pepper, cucumbers, and green onions.
- Serve in individual bowls. If desired, top with sesame seeds, fresh limes, and additional green onions.
- Enjoy!

Make Ahead:

- Pasta can be made several hours ahead. They tend to soak up a lot of the sauce as they sit. If you want to make it the day before, hold back half of the sauce, cover, and chill. Toss with reserved sauce before serving.

16. Carrot sticks with pesto

Prep time: 10 min

Cook time: 20 min

Total time: 30 min

Serving: 4

INGREDIENTS

- Roasted Carrots
- 1 lb. Carrots Scrubbed and rinsed
- 1 Tbsp Olive Oil
- 1/2 Tsp Salt
- Dill Pesto
- 1 1/2 Cup of Carrot Tops De-stemmed and roughly chopped
- 1/2 Cup of Fresh Dill Roughly chopped
- 1/2 Cup of Pecans Roughly chopped
- 1 Clove Garlic Minced
- 1/2 Cup of Olive Oil
- 1/2 Tsp Ground Mustard
- 1 Tbsp Lemon Juice
- 1/2 Tsp Salt

INSRUCTIONS

1. Set oven temperature to 425 degrees. Take the tops off the carrots, wash them, and peel them if you like while the oven is preheating.
2. Place the carrots evenly on a baking sheet and toss with salt and olive oil.
3. To make carrots soft and easy to penetrate with a fork, roast them for 20 minutes. The thickness of your carrots will determine the cooking time, so be sure to check them periodically around the 15-minute point.
4. In a food processor, combine all of the dill pesto ingredients until finely chopped and combined while the carrots roast. Now is the moment to add olive oil if you want a thinner consistency.
5. When the carrots are roasted, serve them warm and top with pesto.

17. Carried broccoli with chili and lemon zest

Prep time: 10 min

Cook time: 20 min

Total time: 30 min

Serving: 4

INGREDIENTS

- Extra-virgin olive oil for cooking
- 1 large head of broccoli, cut into florets (about 5 cups), then cut in half to create a flat base
- Kosher salt
- 2 cloves garlic, sliced
- 1 small shallot, sliced into rings
- 1/4 tsp Chile flakes
- 1 tbsp lemon zest plus 2 tablespoons lemon juice (from 1 lemon)

INSTRUCTIONS

1. Pour 1 tbsp of olive oil into a large pan and set it over medium-high heat. Once the oil is hot, evenly distribute the broccoli and add the flat sides. Season with 1/2 teaspoon of salt. For two minutes, do not stir the broccoli as it cooks. After flipping, heat for another 2–3 minutes or until broccoli is tender-crisp. Set aside the broccoli after transferring it to a platter.
2. Reduce the heat to low and stir in half a tablespoon of olive oil. Toss in the shallot, garlic, and Chile flakes; simmer, stirring often, for 2–3 minutes or until soft. Incorporate the lemon zest and juice after turning off the heat. Stir to blend.
3. Arrange the broccoli on a serving platter and top with the lemon-shallot sauce.

18. Garlic sauteed spinach with pine nuts.

Prep time: 10 min

Cook time: 5 min

Total time: 15 min

Serving: 6

INGREDIENTS

3 pounds spinach, rinsed

2 tsp olive oil

2 tbsp toasted pine nuts

1 tsp minced garlic

Freshly ground black pepper

INSTRUCTIONS

- Rinse the spinach, but make sure the water stays on the leaves. Toss the spinach in a pan and cook until it begins to wilt, approximately 3 minutes over medium-high heat.
- The oil should be heated in a skillet over medium-high heat. After 2 minutes, stir in the garlic, pine nuts, and spinach. Before serving, add pepper.

19. Pumpkin seeds clusters

Prep time: 5 min

Cook time: 45 min

Total time: 50 min

Serving: 6

INGREDIENTS

- 1 cup of pumpkin seeds*
- 2 tsp chili powder
- 1 tsp salt
- 2 tsp maple syrup

INSTRUCTIONS

1. Bring oven temperature up to 275°F. Use cooking paper to line a baking sheet. Combine everything in a medium bowl. Evenly distribute the mixture onto the baking pan. So that they cook into clusters and let the seeds contact just a little. After 35–40 minutes in the oven, let them cool completely before slicing them into clusters. Incorporate it into salads and sandwiches, or enjoy it as a nutritious snack!

20. Jicama carrot and apple salad

Prep time: 2hr

Total time: 2hr

Serving: 3

INGREDIENTS

- 1 large Jicama, peeled and sliced into thin matchsticks
- 2 large Carrots, peeled and sliced into thin matchsticks
- 1 Honeycrisp Apple, sliced into thin matchsticks
- 1 tsp salt
- 2 lemons, juiced and zested
- 4 tbsp olive oil
- 2 tbsp honey
- 2 tsp fresh parsley, chopped

INSTRUCTIONS

2. Place the Jicama, Carrot, and Apple matchsticks in a large mixing bowl, then sprinkle with salt. Toss and blend well, then set aside.
3. In a small mixing bowl, whisk the juice and zest of the lemons, add the olive oil, honey and fresh parsley, and whisk until the mixture gets a little creamy.
4. Pour the lemon and honey dressing over the salad and toss well, ensuring the ingredients are covered well. Cover and place in the refrigerator for at least 2 hours before serving.
5. Serve cold and will keep in the refrigerator for about 5 days.

1. Orange Sorbet

Prep time: 5 min

Cook time: 5 min

Total time: 10 min

Serving: 2

INGREDIENTS

- 300ml orange juice
- 2-star anise
- 100g caster sugar
- Our Most Popular Alternative
- Lemon curd & orange cake

INSTRUCTIONS

1. Toss the sugar, star anise, and orange juice into a saucepan. After the sugar has dissolved, remove the star anise and boil while stirring. Let it cool, then process it in an ice cream maker until it's completely frozen and creamy. (If an ice cream maker isn't available, simply let the liquid cool before pouring it into a freezer-safe container; stir the mixture once an hour to break up any ice crystals.) Freeze until hard.

2. Fruit mousse

Prep time: 10 min

Cook time: 10 min

Total time: 20 min

Serving: 3

INGREDIENTS

1) Prepare an Italian Meringue:

- 8 oz. Sugar
- 2 oz. Water
- 4 oz. Egg Whites
- 1/2 tsp. Cream of Tartar
- 1/2 oz. Sugar

INSTRUCTIONS

1. Gently heat the water and sugar until the temperature reaches 240 degrees Fahrenheit. Soft peaks should be achieved while whipping egg whites, cream of tartar, and 1/2 oz. Sugar. Drizzle 240°F sugar slowly into the beaten egg whites. Whip the mixture with a KitchenAid mixer until it cools. Hold 1/2 for use in the recipe! Keep the leftovers in the fridge when you want to make another mousse.
2. Get the heavy cream to a soft peak by whipping it. Put it in the fridge for later.
3. After 5 minutes, bloom the gelatin in 4 ounces of water. When the water is simmering, add the ingredients and stir until they dissolve.
4. Transfer the fruit purée to a serving dish. Toss in the gelatin mixture and let it chill a little in a bowl of cold water. After that, delicately fold in the Italian meringue. Stir in the whipped topping.
5. Transfer to glasses or prepared molds.

3. Keto almond flour croissants

Prep time: 25 min

Cook time: 25 min

Total time: 50 min

Serving: 4

INGREDIENTS

- ¼ cup of coconut flour
- 2 tbsp powdered Swerve Sweetener (plus more for dusting the croissants)
- ½ tsp xanthan gum
- 1 tsp baking powder
- 6 ounces mozzarella
- 1 large egg
- ⅓ recipe keto almond paste
- 1 tbsp butter, melted
- 1 tbsp sliced almonds broken up a bit with your fingers

INSTRUCTIONS

1. Line a large baking sheet with silicone and heat the oven to 400F. Mount a baking rack to the second-highest setting on your oven.
2. Combine the xanthan gum, baking powder, sweetener, coconut flour, and a medium bowl. Remove off the table.
3. To make the cheese virtually liquid, melt it in a big microwave oven for 30 seconds. Knead the dough in the sized bowl using a rubber spatula after adding the egg and flour combination.

4. Transfer to the baking sheet that has been preheated and keep mixing until a cohesive dough forms. Adding more tablespoons or teaspoons of coconut flour may be necessary if the dough remains sticky.

5. Roll out the dough to a 12-inch shape, then cover with a big waxed or parchment paper sheet. Get a pizza wheel or a big sharp knife and cut it into 8 equal wedges.

6. Separate approximately 1 ½ teaspoons of the almond paste and shape it into a narrow log that is approximately 3 inches in length. Wrap the almond paste securely in the dough, starting at the broad end of one wedge. Seal the seam by pinching it. Make another pass with the leftover dough.

7. Curl the ends of the croissants to make a crescent shape, and place them around the baking sheet. Melt some butter and brush it over the top. Then, press the sliced almonds down firmly. Put it on the oven's designated rack and reduce the heat to 350 degrees Fahrenheit.

8. Cook for 18–25 minutes or until risen and lightly browned. Once removed and cooled, sprinkle with sugar powder.

4. Peach smoothie

Prep time: 5 min

Total time: 5 min

Serving: 2

INGREDIENTS

Peach Yogurt Smoothie (Peach Lassi)

- 1½ cups of peach slices frozen or fresh and peeled
- ¾ cup of Greek yogurt
- ¼ cup of milk. Adjust as needed
- 1 tbsp lemon juice
- 1 tbsp honey or maple syrup; adjust per taste
- 1 Pinch salt
- 1 Pinch of ground cardamom or grated ginger, optional
- Ice cubes
- Fresh mint leaves and peach slices, to decorate

Peach Raspberry Smoothie

- ½ cup of raspberries fresh or frozen
- 2 tbsp honey or maple syrup; adjust per taste
- 1 cup of peach slices frozen or fresh and peeled
- ½ cup of whole milk
- 1 Pinch salt
- Ice cubes optional
- Fresh raspberries, whipped cream, or vanilla ice cream to decorate
- Peach Passion Fruit Drink
- 1 cup of peach slices frozen or fresh and peeled
- 2 tbsp peach jam I use a jam sweetened with fruit juices
- 1 cup of sparkling water. Adjust as needed
- 1 Pinch salt
- 2 passion fruits
- Ice cubes

Peach Coconut Smoothie

- 1½ cups of peach slices frozen or fresh and peeled
- ¾ cup of full-fat coconut milk plus more

- ¼ cup of heavy cream. You can skip this if using full-fat canned coconut milk
- 1 tbsp lemon juice more per taste
- 1 tbsp maple syrup or honey
- 1 tsp natural vanilla extract
- 1 Pinch salt
- Ice cubes or crushed Ice
- Roasted coconut flakes and crushed candied maple pecans to decorate

INSTRUCTIONS

Peach Lassi, a Yogurt Smoothie

- Combine the sliced peaches with the yoghurt, milk, lemon juice, honey, salt, and whichever seasonings you use in a high-speed blender. Whip it until it becomes creamy by using a high-speed blender. Honey and milk or yoghurt can adjust the sweetness and consistency. Serve in large, ice-filled glasses. Put a peach slice on the glass's rim and garnish with mint leaves.
- Make a basic yoghurt smoothie with honey and cover it with the peach lassi, just like the peach raspberry smoothie below. That's one variation.

Raspberry Peach Smoothie

- Combine the raspberries with 1 tablespoon of honey in a food processor. After pureeing the mixture in a food processor, pour it into a small dish and wash the bowl well.
- After that, make a smooth puree by blending peach slices, milk, salt, and 1 tablespoon of honey. Before serving:

- Layer the following ingredients in a chilled glass: half of the peach smoothie, half of the raspberry puree, and then the other half of the peach smoothie and raspberry puree.
- Toss the layers around a little using a whisk stick.
- Before serving, garnish with fresh raspberries.
- Garnish it with some whipped cream or vanilla ice cream to make it more like a peach melba.
- Fruity, Fragrant Peach Soda
- Grind the peach slices, jam, sparkling water, and salt in a blender. Additionally, process until completely smooth. Maintain a pourable yet somewhat thick consistency. Add more jam to taste. Put ⅓ of the mixture onto an ice cube tray and keep it in the freezer for two hours. The peach drink should be refrigerated.
- Spoon the ice cubes into tall, cold glasses when they have cooled. Spoon the peach nectar into each glass.
- Segment the passion fruit lengthwise. Divide the peach into three equal parts and remove the pulp. Add the pulp to the peach drink and gently mix. Make decorative wedges out of the leftover passion fruit.
- Pulp some passion fruit and mix it in with the other ingredients for a different twist.

Coconut Peach Smoothie

- Ingredients for the blended drink include sliced peaches, coconut milk, cream, lemon juice, maple syrup, vanilla essence, salt, and four cubes of Ice. Mix till you get a thick, pourable consistency. To taste, add maple syrup for sweetness and coconut milk for consistency.

- Fill up to three-quarters of the glasses with the peach coconut smoothie once they are cooled. Incorporate a few chopped maple pecans and a small amount of coconut milk. Layer again twice more. When serving, garnish with toasted coconut flakes and use a wide straw for smoothies.
- Make it your own by blending some pineapple pieces with the peaches.

5. Banana chocolate bites

Prep time: 15 min

Additional time: 1hr

Total time: 1hr 15 min

Serving: 4

INGREDIENTS

- 2 medium bananas
- 1 ½ ounces special dark chocolate pieces (about 1/3 cup)

INSTRUCITONS

1. Chop bananas. Peel the bananas and cut them into half-inch slices. Spread waxed paper or parchment paper on a cooking sheet. On the baking sheet, place the banana slices close together in one layer.
2. The best way to melt chocolate is in a heavy pot set over low heat. Fill a tiny, resealable plastic bag with the melted chocolate. Close the bag and cut off a little corner. Top sliced bananas with melted chocolate.

Once frozen, cover and freeze for another hour or two.

3. Four tiny resealable freezer bags or containers will do the trick for dividing the banana chunks. Keep in the freezer for a maximum of three days.

6. Lemon tart

Prep time: 10 min

Cook time: 15 min

Total time: 25 min

Serving: 4

INGREDIENTS

- 1 sweet tart crust (or homemade pie crust, or store-bought 23cm / 9" sweet pie or tart crust)
- LEMON TART FILLING:
- 1 tbsp lemon zest (1 lemon's worth)
- 1/2 cup of lemon juice (from 1 – 2 lemons)
- 3/4 cup of white sugar
- 12 tbsp / 170g unsalted butter, cut into 1cm (1/2") cubes
- 3 whole eggs large
- 3 egg yolks (from large-size eggs)

INSTRUCTIONS

- TART CRUST: Blind bake the unfilled tart crust as directed in the attached recipe. To avoid sogginess, let it cool completely before filling.

Filling for Lemon Tarts:

- Warm up the oven: Heat the oven to 180 degrees Celsius (350 Fahrenheit; 160 degrees Celsius fan).

- Mix the items in a bowl. Whisk together all of the ingredients in a medium saucepan.
- Simmer to thicken: Set the saucepan over medium-low heat on the stove. To prevent the butter from splitting, whisk continuously, particularly when it melts. It should take around 5 minutes, but depending on stove strength, saucepan heat retention, etc., it might take longer to thicken the mixture to the point that it mounds (holds its form temporarily) on the surface when dolloped. Be sure to keep stirring throughout this time.
- Thickness guidance may be found in the movie and images. The Filling won't set until you keep it on the heat until it thickens.
- Use a fine mesh strainer to put the mixture to a bowl.
- Pour filling into a tart shell and use an offset spatula to smooth the surface of the Filling.
- Pop in the oven and cook for five minutes. You can still feel the custard's softness when you touch it, but it won't be liquid. Once chilled, it will firm even more, making it easy to slice.
- Let the tart cool completely so it can firm before cutting it into serving pieces. The lemon pie is complemented beautifully with crème fraiche, whipped cream, or vanilla ice cream, which are rich, thick creams with a hint of acidity.
- Garnish with lemon slices, edible flowers, and raspberries if you want. Another option is to garnish with icing sugar or pipe on whipped cream.

7. Baked apple with orange

Prep time: 10 min

Total time: 10 min

Serving: 2

INGREDIENTS

- 25g Flora Proactive Buttery
- 2 cooking apples
- 30g fresh root ginger finely chopped
- 4 tbsp water
- 1 orange zested
- 1/4 tsp ground ginger
- 1 tbsp runny honey
- 55g dates finely chopped

INSTRUCTIONS

1. Set oven temperature to 200°C (fan oven 180°C, gas mark 6).
2. Before using an apple corer to extract the core and pips, delicately score the apples around the core with a sharp knife. Arrange in a baking dish.
3. Stuff the apples' centers with a combination of dates and raw ginger. Pour the water into the bowl. To get a soft and cooked consistency, bake for 30 to 35 minutes.
4. Add the orange zest, ground ginger, honey, and Flora Proactive spread as you wait.
5. When the apples are done, top them with the Flora Proactive spread that has been flavored and let it melt.

8. Coconut flour muffins

Prep time: 10 min

Cook time: 20 min

Total time: 30 min

Serving: 10

INGREDIENTS

- ¾ cup of coconut flour
- 1 tsp baking powder
- ¼ tsp sea salt
- 4 large eggs
- ½ cup of canned coconut milk (the liquid only) or unsweetened almond milk
- ½ cup of maple syrup
- ½ tsp vanilla extract
- ¾ cup of blueberries, plus more for topping

INSTRUCTIONS

1. Set oven temperature to 400°F. In a muffin pan, lay out ten cupcake liners, either paper or silicone.
2. Whisk the salt, baking soda, and coconut flour in a small bowl.
3. Coconut flour, baking soda, and salt are all combined in a little basin.
4. Combine the eggs, coconut milk, maple syrup, and vanilla extract in an average-sized bowl and whisk until well combined.
5. Whisk together the eggs, coconut milk, maple syrup, and vanilla seed in a medium-sized bowl.
6. After adding the dry ingredients to the basin containing the wet ones, stir until barely mixed. The coconut flour needs around five minutes to soak up the liquid, so let the mixture sit for that long.
7. Combining the dry ingredients with the liquid ones.
8. Carefully incorporate the blueberries into the mixture, then distribute it evenly among ten muffin pans.
9. Incorporating freshly picked blueberries into the muffin mixture.
10. After inserting a toothpick into the middle of the muffin, bake for 18 to 20 minutes or until it emerges clean.
11. Baked muffins in a 6-muffin pan.
12. The muffins should be allowed to cool in the pan for around 5 minutes before being removed and allowed to cool entirely on a wire rack.
13. Keep for three to four days at room temperature or sealed in the fridge for up to a week. Another option is to store it in the freezer for up to three months.

9. Fruit and nuts with seeds

Prep time: 2hr 10 min

Total time: 2hr 10 min

Serving: 2

INGREDIENTS

- 2 kiwis
- 1 banana
- 4 tbsp walnuts
- 1/2 cup of coconut milk
- 2 tbsp chia seeds
- 1/4 cup pomegranate seeds
- 1 moambe
- 4 tbsp pistachios
- 1 tbsp honey

INSTRUCTIONS

1. First, get the dressing ready.
2. Toss the chia seeds, honey, and coconut milk into a bowl. Refrain from stirring for at least two hours. Your salad will have a rich dressing thanks to this.
3. Step 2: Mince the nutmeg and fruit.
4. Now, you should peel and finely dice all the fruits. Transfer to a basin. In addition, combine the fruits with the coarsely chopped nuts.
5. Third, drizzle with the dressing and enjoy!
6. Add the chia seed dressing to the salad and gently toss to combine. Your chia salad with fruit and nuts is done when you are.

10. Nut and fruit roll

Prep time: 10 min

Cook time: 5 min

Total time: 15 min

Serving: 2

INGREDIENTS

- Almonds slivered - 1/4 cup
- Cashews -1/4 cup
- Pistachios -1/4 cup
- Walnuts - 1/4 cup
- Pumpkin seeds -1/4 cup
- Goji Berries - 1/4 cup
- Cranberries - 1/4 cup
- Raisins - 1/4 cup
- Figs - 1/2 cup
- Dates - 2 cups (pitted)
- Sesame seeds - 1/2 cup as topping (roasted)
- Cling wrap - optional

INSTRUCTIONS

1. First, use a knife to roughly chop the nuts and dried fruits individually. In increments of a few, I blended the dates in my blender.
2. While the pumpkin seeds release their oil, dry roast the nuts in a large skillet over medium heat. Get it out of the oven.
3. Step 3: Dry roast all dried fruits (except the dates) in the same skillet for a minute or two. Then, after another two minutes of mixing, add the dates. Toss in all the nuts and mix thoroughly.
4. Once it reaches room temperature, take it from the stove and roll it into a log. Place it on a tray and sprinkle toasted sesame seeds on top to stick.
5. Step 5: Securely wrap in cling wrap and chill to set for at least two hours. Serve at room temperature after slicing. Put it somewhere airtight or vacuum-sealed to keep it fresh.

11. Cottage cheese baked raisins

Prep time: 15 min

Cook time: 35 min

Total time: 50 min

Serving: 4

INGREDIENTS

- cottage cheese - 2 lb. (1 kg)
- eggs - 5
- sugar - 1 cup
- flour - 5 tbsp
- lemons - 1
- raising agent - 1/2 tsp

- cream - 4/5 cup (200 g)
- raisins - 3.5 oz (100 g) large
- measures
- CASSEROLE

INSTRUCTIONS

1. Whisk the cottage cheese, eggs, and sugar with the cream in an appropriate deep bowl. Gradually incorporate the sifted flour, rising agent, and finely grated lemon peel into the mixture.
2. Blend the ingredients. Rinse raisins in hot water and then include them in other recipes. Remix until evenly distributed.
3. After greasing the baking dish, transfer the mixture to the oven and cook for approx. 35 minutes at 360°F (180°C).

12. Almond cookies

Prep time: 10 min

Cook time: 15 min

Total time: 25 min

Serving: 12

INGREDIENTS

For the egg wash:

- 2 tbsp (30 ml) water
- 1 egg
- For the cookie:
- 1 1/2 cups of (350 ml) all-purpose flour
- 3/4 cup of (180 ml) sugar
- 1/2 tsp (2.5 ml) baking soda
- 1/2 tsp (2.5 ml) salt
- 1 cup of (240 ml) butter, room temperature
- 1 egg

- 1 tsp (5 ml) almond extract

INSTRUCTIONS:

1. Preheat the oven to 325 grades Fahrenheit (160 degrees Celsius).
2. The egg wash is made by mixing equal water with one egg.
3. Whisk the flour, sugar with baking soda, and salt for the cookie in a medium bowl.
4. Gradually add the butter to the dry ingredients while mixing with a hand mixer.
5. Just before combining, add the egg and almond essence.
6. Shape dough into balls and space them two inches on an ungreased baking sheet. Get the balls flat by pressing down hard.
7. Bake for fifteen minutes after lightly brushing with egg wash.
8. Cool before serving after removing from oven.

13. Oat bars with nuts and dried fruit

Prep time: 10 min

Cook time: 25 min

Total time; 35 min

Serving: 20

INGREDIENTS

Dry Ingredients

- 3/4 cup of rolled oats
- 1/2 cup of pecans, chopped
- 1/2 cup of finely shredded unsweetened coconut
- 1/2 cup of dried cranberries
- 1/4 cup of whole wheat flour
- 2 tbsp chia seeds
- 1/2 tsp salt, I use Himalayan salt

- 1/2 tsp ground cinnamon
- 1/4 tsp baking powder
- 1/4 tsp baking soda

Wet Ingredients

- 2 large eggs at room temperature
- 2 tbsp melted coconut oil
- 1/2 cup of creamy peanut butter
- 1/4 cup of unpasteurized honey
- 1/2 tsp pure vanilla extract
- Optional
- 16-20 pecan halves, to decorate

INSTRUCTIONS

1. Turn the oven on high heat (350°F). Set aside a 9-inch baking pan that has been greased and lined with parchment paper.
2. Toss the dry ingredients into a large basin and stir with a whisk or fork until well-mixed.
3. Whisk the wet ingredients in a separate smaller bowl until smooth and well blended; add the dry elements and stir with a rubber spatula until completely incorporated.
4. After preparing the pan, transfer the dough and spread it out evenly. If desired, press pecan halves lightly over the top.
5. After inserting a toothpick into the middle of the cake, bake it for another 23–25 minutes or until it turns a beautiful golden brown on top.
6. After an hour of chilling on a cooling rack, remove the pan from the bars and cut it into sixteen to twenty bars.
7. The bars can be kept for up to a week if stored in an airtight container in a cool, dry area.

14. Tiramisu shots

Prep time: 10 min

Additional time: 2hr

Total time: 2hr 10 min

Serving: 4

INGREDIENTS

- 250 gm whipping cream
- 200 gm powdered sugar
- 1/4 cup of espresso coffee
- ladyfinger biscuit as required
- 200 gm mascarpone cheese
- 1 tsp vanilla extract
- 2 tbsp coffee liqueur
- 1 tbsp cocoa powder

INSTRUCTIONS

- First, whisk the cream until foamy.
- A bowl and a hand mixer fitted with the whisk attachment should whip the cream at medium speed.
- Second, combine the sugar and vanilla essence.
- While beating, gradually add sugar and vanilla extract until stiff peaks develop.
- Third, incorporate the mascarpone cheese.
- Combine with the mascarpone cheese by mixing briefly. Temporarily set aside.
- Fourth, whip up a coffee mixture.
- In a bowl, combine the coffee and coffee liqueur. Combine to form a mixture.
- Fifth, Build the Tiramisu Layers
- Just moisten the ladyfinger cookies by dipping them in the coffee, then arrange them in a single layer on the base of a glass dish. Disperse

half of the mascarpone mixture evenly over the surface. Layer the ladyfingers cookies again with the dipping sauce. To make another layer, use the leftover mascarpone cream.

- Final Garnishing Step 6
- Coat with cocoa powder and decorate with cut fruits of your choosing. Put in the fridge for a minimum of two to three hours.
- Step 7: All Set to Be Offered
- Best enjoyed cold.

15. Brule orange

Prep time: 10 min

Cook time: 35 min

Total time: 45 min

Serving: 5

INGREDIENTS

- 5 egg yolks
- 1 cup of sugar
- 3 cups heavy whipping cream
- Zest of 1 orange
- 2 tsp. vanilla extract
- ½ tsp. salt
- Mint, raspberries & orange slices for serving

INSTRUCTIONS

1. Get your oven hot, about 325°F.
2. Whisk the egg yolks and 1/4 cup of sugar with a whisk. Put aside.
3. In a small saucepan, bring the water to a boil. This is what the water bath will use.
4. In a saucepan, combine the cream with the salt and orange zest. Once it reaches a simmer, take it off the heat. Add the vanilla extract and mix well.
5. Gently stir 1 cup of the heated cream to the egg yolk and sugar mixture. Pour it slowly while whisking constantly. The eggs will be scrambled, and the lovely cream will be ruined if you add too much too quickly. While whisking constantly, slowly pour in the remaining cream.
6. Fill a baking pan that is one to two inches deep with 5 individual ramekins. Fill the baking pan halfway with boiling water, then add the ramekins.
7. Spoon half an inch of cream into each ramekin. Put in the oven and cook for half an hour.
8. At the 30-minute mark, give the crème Brulé a taste. The center should be positioned just slightly.
9. After removing it from the oven, let it cool on a wire rack for at least one hour. Wrap in plastic and refrigerate for at least three hours after the first hour.
10. Take it out of the fridge and sprinkle the remaining sugar on top after three hours.
11. Finish by caramelizing the sugar using a cooking torch. To avoid burning the sugar, keep the flame moving. In the absence of an adult, broil the food in the oven.
12. Arrange some sliced oranges, fresh berries, and a mint leaf on top. Break open that sugar and savor it!

16. Broiled stone fruit

Prep time: 10 min

Cook time: 25 min

Total time: 35 min

Serving: 4

INGREDIENTS

Soft Serve:

- 3 frozen bananas
- 2 cups Almond Breeze Almond milk Vanilla
- 1 tsp ground cinnamon
- **1 tsp ground cardamom**

Stone Fruit:

- 2 plums, halved and pitted
- 2 nectarines, halved and pitted
- ⅛ cup of sugar
- 2 tbsp apple cider
- Chia seeds for garnish
- Fresh blueberries for garnish

INSTRUCTIONS

1. After arranging the fruit on a baking dish with the sliced side facing up, drizzle with cider. After 17 minutes in a preheated oven at 425 degrees F, sprinkle with sugar and broil to finish browning.
2. Blend all ingredients until smooth to produce a soft serve. If you want it more scoopable, put it in the freezer for an hour before serving or beneath the fruit.
3. Add blueberries and chia seeds as a garnish.

17. Kamut porridge

Prep time: 20 min

Cook time: 40 min

Total time: 1hr

Serving: 4

INGREDIENTS

- 1 cup of Kamut uncooked
- 2 tbsp olive oil
- 1 cup of chopped sweet onion
- 3 cloves garlic minced
- 1 ½ cups of chopped carrots
- 2 cups of kale chopped into bite-sized pieces
- 1 cup of roasted pumpkin seeds
- juice of 1 fresh lemon
- 3 green onions chopped

INSTRUCTIONS

1. Following your chosen technique from the list above, cook the kamut in vegetable broth. Cubes of Not Chicken Broth were what I used.
2. In a giant skillet, heat the oil over medium heat. With the onions softening, add the carrots and garlic and simmer for another 7 minutes, stirring occasionally.
3. Toss in the kale and continue cooking for another four to five minutes or until it reaches a deep, dark green colour.
4. Combine the cooked kamut with the greens, pumpkin seeds, and lemon juice in a big bowl. Before serving, garnish with green onions.

18. Coconut pudding cloud

Cook time: 15 min

Additional time: 4hr

Total time: 4hr 15 min

Serving: 6

INGREDIENTS

- 6 tbsp cornstarch
- 1/4 tsp salt
- 1-1/2 cups of whole milk, divided use
- 1-1/2 cups of coconut milk
- 1 cup of granulated sugar
- 1/2 to 1 tsp coconut extract
- Optional garnish: shredded coconut

INSTRUCTIONS

1. Combine the cornstarch and salt in a medium bowl and whisk to combine. Pour in half a cup of milk gradually while whisking to combine.
2. In a 2-quart pot, combine the sugar, coconut milk, and the 1 cup of milk set aside. While stirring constantly, simmer over medium heat and cook until the sugar dissolves. Add cornstarch mixture slowly while stirring continually until the liquid becomes extremely thick, which should take around 5 to 6 minutes. Turn the heat off. Then, after another minute of stirring, add coconut essence according to taste. Give it another 10 to 15 minutes to cool.
3. Divide the custard among six 3/4-cup serving dishes. Allow 4 to 6 hours in the fridge for the mixture to cool and solidify. Shredded coconut can be used as a garnish if preferred.

19. Pineapple frozen yoghurt

Prep time: 10 min

Total time: 10 min

Serving: 1

INGREDIENTS

- 2 cups of frozen pineapple
- 1/4 cup of Greek yoghurt plain or vanilla

INSTRUCTIONS

1. Combine the frozen pineapple and yoghurt in a food processor or high-speed blender until smooth. Scrape down the edges if necessary.
2. Fill a dish with it and savor it. It is recommended to have this dessert immediately after serving.

20. Blueberry lemon cupcake

Prep time; 20 min

Cook time: 20 min

Cooking time: 2hr

Total time: 2hr 40 min

Serving: 15

INGREDIENTS

- 1 and 1/2 cups (188g) all-purpose flour (spooned & levelled)
- 2 tsp baking powder
- 1/2 tsp salt
- 1/2 cup of (8 Tbsp; 113g) unsalted butter, softened to room temperature
- 1 cup of (200g) granulated sugar
- 1 tbsp lemon zest
- 2 large eggs at room temperature
- 1 and 1/2 teaspoons pure vanilla extract

- 1/2 cup of (120ml) whole milk or buttermilk at room temperature
- 1/4 cup of (60ml) fresh lemon juice
- 1 cup of (140g) fresh or frozen blueberries, tossed in 1 Tablespoon flour
- Cream Cheese Frosting
- 8 ounces (226g) full-fat brick cream cheese, softened to room temperature
- 1/4 cup (4 Tbsp; 56g) unsalted butter, softened to room temperature
- 2 cups of (240g) confectioners' sugar
- 1 tsp pure vanilla extract
- pinch salt
- optional: lemon slices and extra blueberries for garnish

INSTRUCTIONS

- Make sure the oven is preheated to 350°F (177°C). Put cupcake liners in a muffin pan that holds 12 cups. You will have an extra batch of cupcakes because this recipe makes around 15 of them.
- Retrieve the batter: In a large bowl, whisk together the flour, baking soda, and salt. Put aside.
- Cream the butter, sugar, and lemon zest in a giant basin using a paddle attachment or a medium-high-held handheld mixer for about 2 minutes. You may need to scrape the bowl's sides and bottom occasionally. Pour the eggs and vanilla extract and beat quickly once mixed, which should take around a minute. You may need to scrape the bowl's sides and bottom occasionally. Toss in the dry ingredients, then gradually add the milk and lemon juice while mixing quickly. Mix until barely mixed.

After the blueberries have been floured, fold them in. Stir gently.

- Spoon the batter into the liners, filling those two-thirds to the top to prevent any spillage. Stick a toothpick into the middle and bake for 18 to 21 minutes to test doneness. Bake thirty to forty-six miniature cupcakes at the same temperature for eleven to thirteen minutes. Before icing, make sure the cupcakes have cooled entirely.

Whip up the frosting:

- Mix up the cream cheese and butter in a large basin.
- Use a stand mixer with a whisk to beat until smooth, which should take approximately 2 minutes.
- After 30 seconds on low speed, add salt, vanilla extract, and confectioners' sugar; continue beating for 2 minutes on medium-high speed.
- Fix seasoning with a pinch of salt and add more if needed.
- Put this frosting in the fridge for at least 20 minutes before you frost complicated patterns.
- Once the cupcakes have cooled, frost them and, if you choose, top them with a garnish. Another option would be to use a little icing spatula. To help set the icing, refrigerate the frosted cupcakes uncovered for at least 20 minutes before serving.
- Keep any unused cupcakes covered in the fridge for up to five days. The use of a cupcake container facilitates both transportation and storage.